Sex positions for Couples

Sexual beginner's guide for men and women. Use your sexuality energy to explore your fantasy. Tips for dominant positions that will turn your sex life

Alexia Reid

Table of Contents

Introduction

Thank you for downloading this book on Sex for Couples. The chapters in this book will give you an analysis of styles, tips, and the gist of giving your partner mind-blowing intimacy and orgasms. The first chapter the book introduces sex and its basics. The chapter discusses the importance of sex in a couple's life, the stimulants of sex. You will learn more about what arouses your partner. The chapter further looks at sex communication. You will understand why it is important for a great intimate connection. Finally, the chapter discusses sexual compatibility.

In chapter two, the book dives in to discuss the stimulants of sexual intercourse. Remember before you get into the mind bowing positions you need to be well aroused and that dick better is erect to do the did. The book discusses oral sex, oral-anal sex, foreplay, fingering, and sex toys. Get to understand how all these techniques contribute to your sex life as a couple. The third chapter discusses sex positions. The book is going to expound on the best sex positions that are going to lead you to an immense orgasm. Also if you do not have a bucket list of sex positions to try, you will find some right in this book. Still, in the same chapter, get to know the importance of sex positions. The fourth chapter discusses sexual health. The book expounds on the importance of sexual health, physical intimacy, and anal sex. Dive in to read more. The fifth chapter discusses sexual fantasy. You have a sex fantasy that you would love to try. Get to know more on the fetish. Also, what if you do not like the sexual fetish of your partner? The book explains how to handle such a situation.

Finally, the sixth chapter looks at the sex tips. The book details what to do to improve your sexual libido. Further, there is a discussion on giving your partner an erotic massage and concludes with giving you like a couple of sex tips to improve your sex life.

I would like to thank you for choosing this book amid plenty of similar books in the market. Every effort was made to ensure it is full of as much useful information as possible, please enjoy! Remember to leave a review on Amazon!

Chapter 1

Introduction to sex

Sex to distinct individuals implies different things. It is, more than anything, a natural and healthy activity. This is something many individuals appreciate and find valuable even though they generate significance in distinct ways. Even if you're straight, gay, lesbian, bisexual, you have all the right to determine what sex means to you. The sexual act is defined as the insertion of the penis in the vagina and thrusting for pleasure or reproduction. There are also other types of intercourse which include; Anal sex, the penetration through the anus, Oral sex which is penetration through the mouth or female genitals, fingering involves penetration using fingers and finally we have use of dildos which is the toys used for pleasure. All these forms are physical and contribute to emotional pleasure in a person. The book shall dive more into this, but first, let us look at what stimulates sex.

Sex is stimulated by different acts and initiatives by a partner. It is also to be noted that, you as an individual has weak points and stimulants that turn you on automatically. Some of the stimulants are;

Sex positions-there are sex positions that are hot and turn you and your partner on for intercourse

Foreplay-which happens before intercourse and leads to sexual arousal, this maybe kissing, touching or talking dirty

Sex toy-Use of sex toys may be a stimulator for different individuals

Is sex real intimacy

Sex is not a proof of love. You may find a potential partner who is interested in you, but first, he insists that you need to have sex to bond. My dear that is a myth, to say that sex leads to intimacy. To break this down, you need to be aware that sex can be the most amazing and profound expression of love. You will, however, be deceiving yourself if you agree that sex is a proof of love. Being used has become so common in our society, in that men ask for sex as proof of your love for them. A lot of women have fallen into this trap and left crying because the men vanished, some left pregnant and others in the thirst of intimacy. This can be termed as abuse of love, where some individuals deceive to fill the void that they have on the inside. This is because there is taking advantage of the desire to be loved and physical intimacy for every human being. Let us take a case study of Pete and Stella. After marriage, Stella was sure that, despite their emotional distance sex would solve that. This is because she had watched many movies where relationships blossomed after sex. This theory was false because Pete never connected even after sex. The bond was nowhere to be found. What you should know as a couple is that real intimacy is not fueled by sex. We ought to analyze that, when two people are said to become one, it was more than just sex and physical intimacy. Many couples stay in the same household, have sex, but are lonely and hearts apart because there is no intimate connection. This is because, sex does not bring intimacy but rather, you get intimate first and sex is the outlet. You will enjoy the results, of using sex as an expression of the intimate bond that you have created. No matter how much attraction and interest you have in someone, if you do not have a connection before sexual intercourse, do not deceive yourself that it will magically happen after. Where there is real intimacy, an individual feels recognized. We feel alive like we have been found, where there is real intimacy like it is at last somebody took the time to look into the deepest recesses of our heart and found us there. Until then, we will feel passed over and overlooked like we are transparent until we experience real intimacy. Tragically, we can pass up closeness that can make us and someone else feel known when we foreordain what we figure we should see when we analyze their life, heart, character, and soul. At the point when this occurs, we will attempt to shape and cause them into who we to accept they ought to be. Therefore, we are blinded to their great characteristics and love and closeness diminish. For example, when I was dating, one of my mentors advised me that I should not focus on what my partner is not because I will miss on the best thing that they bring. With that, I got a lesson that, ignoring the positive things about a person, we lose the intimacy that is meant to connect us for the better. What you should know is that real intimacy starts with you. This is how you build real intimacy. In addition to accepting another person just how they are, this does not call you to accept abuse, once you know yourself that is when real intimacy begins. Intimacy symbolizes the other person getting to the inside of you and connecting. So, that would not be possible if you do not know yourself. You have to be self-aware of you before you let someone else have a piece of your inner you. Otherwise, if you let other people define you, you are bound to manipulation. Strive to be connected to your own heart. While you find someone, do not open and allow them in immediately, take your time to know their intention and open up as you develop trust. Intimacy with your creator is the most amazing. Connect with him and he will allow you to know yourself better and in turn, find real intimacy with your partner.

Importance of sex for couples

Sex is necessary for couples as an expression for intimacy and other great health reasons. It is part and parcel of your life. You do not just have sex for reproduction but also pleasure and happiness. You may not know this, but sex brings a lot of health benefits in your life ranging from mental, emotional, physical, social and psychological benefits. Sexual health stems to more than seeing it as a threat to unwanted pregnancy and diseases. This book shall focus on the health benefits and the alternatives to make your sex life mind-blowing.

Let us have a look at the importance of sex.

Health benefits for your body

There has been numerous research that states that sex can be a beneficial cardiovascular light exercise for men and women. This is because it has been found to cause calorie burn (Who wouldn't want some calories gone through pleasure), It lowers blood pressure, strengthens muscles, heart health improves, minimizes the risk of suffering from stroke, hypertension, and heart disease, and most of all it contributes in increasing your libido. Individuals with healthy sex lives strive to practice more often and have healthier eating habits than those who have less unhealthy sexual activity. Physical exercise can also enhance general sexual output.

Developing a strong immunity system

Sexual intercourse as been proven to contribute to a strong immune system. A study conducted among the couples in romantic relationships with one measure of having frequent sex that is once to twice a week, proved that their saliva had more immunoglobulin A. those who had sex less that is no sex in a week had less Immunoglobulin A (IgA). Presence of IgA antibody is important because it has a role of preventing illnesses and tops at defending human papilloma virus (HPV). However, the study showed that the IgA of the couples who had sex more than three times a week was the same as those who had infrequent sex. Here is why. Research has proven that stress and anxiety can rub off the positive effects of sex in a person.

Sleeping better

When you experience an orgasm, there is a love hormone released from your body called oxytocin and endorphins. These hormones are sedative to sleep. You all know that good sleep is beneficial. Therefore, due to this, your immune system grows stronger, you feel more relaxed, you get energized and a long life span.

Migraine healing

More research shows that having fulfilling sex brings with it healing from migraines. For the people were suffering from migraines; 70 percent were completely healed, over 60 percent recorded great development while having a migraine. Generally of the couple who were sexually active, the study showed that they were relieved of the migraine.

Benefits to mental health

Did you know that your mental health is also improved through sexual intercourse? Sex brings with it great emotional and psychological benefits. Sex has been found to relieve stress, bring down anxiety and also increase happiness. The benefits that sex brings to your mental health include the following;

There is an increase in trust, intimacy, and love in your relationships, you will feel your mental stability state, you will be alert and able to identify and perceive emotions, you will be mature emotionally. Older couples between 50-60 who are sexually active, are found to be less stressed and have a good memory. They also have a lower level of getting depressed and lonely.

Boosts your confidence

You'll be amazed to note that, having good sex with your partner will make you look younger and have high self-esteem. This is caused by the release of a hormone called estrogen. There is a close relationship between active sex life and looking way younger. You are also able and confident to discuss your sexual awareness comfortably.

Improves your social abilities

Remember the oxytocin hormone (the love hormone), it's beneficial as it helps you have a strong connection with your partner. The hormone also contributes to your having great relationships with your friends and social circle. As a couple, you will be satisfied in your relationship if you both satisfy the individual sexual goals. You will find a lot of development after having the ability to communicate your sexual desires to your partner. This is because sex is not about submitting to the desires of your partner but also getting your desires fulfilled. There is satisfaction in a relationship when desires are met. Your mouth may be wide open now, because you are wondering how to communicate to your partner about your sexual desires, Maybe in fear that he will judge you or view you differently. Worry not because this book will show you how. Keep reading.

What is the benefit of sex to male and female gender

Women

Fulfilling sex for women may be significant in different ways. An orgasm helps you release natural pain-relieving chemicals and also increases the blood flow. Sex helps you reduce menstrual cramping, brings out more vaginal lubrication, helps you have bladder control, strong pelvic muscles, improves fertility and also incontinence reduction.

Men

Good sex for men reveals that they will be less likely to get prostate cancer. Men who have 4-7 ejaculations a week record a less likelihood of being diagnosed with prostate cancer before age 70. Also, sex for men reduces the mortality rate. Men who ejaculate quite often have 50 percent less risk of dying early.

Final take

As we conclude the importance of sex in your life, it is to be noted that, sex is an important activity for your well being. The mind-blowing orgasms that you get are very important for bonding. You have also realized the immense benefits such as the reduced danger of heart disease, high self-esteem, and much more come as a result of having satisfying sex in your relationship. This is not to mean that the celibate people are in danger. The pleasurable effect that one gets during sex can also be compared with exercising, having a pet, the good social circle of friends. Therefore, sex is among the many types of ways of developing your life quality. It is also the main subject of this book. Therefore, if sex is part of your life, it is advisable to take charge and express your desires to have a satisfying sex life.

Sex Communication

Sex communication is very important while in a serious relationship. Research shows that only 9 % of couples who never communicate about sex are happy. Therefore, your sexual satisfaction could culminate into your lack of communication. Most of the time you may assume that your partner is fine because they do not talk, while on the other hand, you may think that he/she never listens and is not concerned. You need to be aware that the assumption does not solve problems. You cannot assume that your partner can tell your issue and solve it. You have to communicate. Being indirect with fear will also not get you the sex of your life. We are going to look at how you can communicate well about sex without feeling left out or sidelined or judged.

Here are the tips for communicating about sex with your partner.

Be positive and humble

It is to be noted that as a couple, good communication etiquette, especially with intimate matters, is paramount. Therefore, when you decide to engage with sex communication, be sure not to seem or come out as a critique. Darling, if you do this, the communication will end even before it amounts to anything meaningful. Can I say it may end faster than your shortest quickie? Now, brace yourself in a calm and emotionally stable way ready to talk. Talking in a way such as,' you don't kiss me passionately, you are rough, I don't get satisfied,' is going to make your partner resentful and do less of that. This is because they have felt attacked. You can instead use statements such as, 'The make out in the car last week was mind-blowing,' 'The kiss you gave me last night was passionate, I'd love more of that,' this is going to make your partner strive more to ensure they get the best price. Tell them in a good way how you like your sex served, touch me here, kiss me like this, I get turned on when you speak dirty...and much more. Most of the time, you may feel ashamed about your body as a man or a woman. Therefore, adding the critique tone while communicating will only make the problem worse. Could be the man is already worried about satisfying you because he thinks he is not fit enough, or as a man your woman is worried because she does not have a nice figure. Therefore, being positive and kind with words as well as assuring that all is well and the communication will make it better is a great move.

Communicating well will also lead to being creative in new ways to express love to each other.

Patience

The fact is that having a conversation about sex may not be so comfortable. Not every individual is sexually confident. Some are conservative and were not brought up to enjoy sex and realize the pleasure that it comes with. Therefore, if you or your partner are anywhere near this scenario, you must become patient. Go step by step and communicate about your feelings towards sex, and the perceptions that you have inclined in yourself. Further, be open about what you feel and what both of you feel. If one of you is experienced, you need to be patient with the newbie. You don't want to be subjected to too much or have a lot of expectation towards your partner when indeed you have not communicated. The conversation will bring closure and help you work out your relationship in a secure way.

Don't personalize it

If you are having some issues in your sex life, it would be prudent to know that, you or your partner is not the cause. For instance, it is not that they do not wish to take you to cloud nine. You should be aware that factors such as stress, anxiety, being broke; embarrassment can lead to a low sex drive. Therefore, your partner not performing fully does not mean that he/she does not find you hot and amazing anymore. You also cannot conclude that your sex life sucks, but it's rather a matter of the situational factors that are there at the moment. In the moments that you are not interested in having sex, you should find good ways to communicate about it. No, you will not be faking migraines or you being tired from work. Gently let your partner get the knowledge of your fears. Maybe you could also come up with a schedule. This will help in preparing your partner that indeed sex is happening tonight and avoid leaving the other person horny or wet, without notice.

Empathy

It is a requirement that you understand the point where your partner is coming from. Communication will need for you as a couple to talk about what feels awkward, good and safe as well as what doesn't and how to improve it. If the solutions require therapy may be due to past experiences, you should support your partner and both attend therapy. This is because as a couple, you are now one and should solve things together. Do not judge. This will lead to good sex, where you make your sex life accommodative of everyone's desires. For instance, you may want sex thrice a week while your partner wants it once a week. You may feel frustrated that your needs are not being met and that your partner is not concerned. If this is not properly discussed, it may lead to cheating and also relationship breaks up. However, you may need to discuss other ways that your partner may be interested during the week such as touching and massages. Initiate them and get the connections, soon or later they will be aroused and satisfied to negotiate another day of sex. And bam, you have two days of sex in a week. What a good compromise. This teaches you that, you should not always jump into conclusions of what is negative, but look at how many solutions you may be blocking in your love relationship.

Communication I art that you can learn with time. More so, sex communication is as important in your relationship as financial talk. Take the initiative and begin to have that bedroom conversation.

Now, as much as we are getting good sex. You should ask yourself, is sex always good? Do we have bad sex? Well, let's dig in.

Sexual questions

Is there a thing like bad sex

Yes, there is something like bad sex. However, at the end of this book, you will have solutions to getting amazing mind-blowing sex and orgasms. It is the hope of every couple and everyone in general to have great sex. But just as we make abrupt bad decisions, an instance of bad sex is normal but solvable. Here are some ouch moments that you can say sex was bad.

Sex for the first time

Looking back now, you may say that losing your virginity wasn't bad, but in reality, the moment was awful. When you are having sex for the first time, it is unfulfilling, painful and you may not tell when it will ever be smooth and heavenly. It involves a lot of pushing and maybe screaming. It is awkward for the experienced one and more awful for the first-timer. Probably, a guy may not know how to thrust well, he may cum fast and get tired easily. He may also not know where to touch and what to do in foreplay. I can confidently tell you that, they're nothing like good first-time sex. It also depends on where you are having your first-time sex. It is worse if it's in the car, kitchen table or floor. If a bed is not comfortable, the floor or car must be the worst. I guess you cannot forget your first-time sex. That can very well be regarded as bad sex.

Nod off sex

This is an awkward situation where you may be at the middle of boring sexual experience and all of a sudden you nod off. You start fantasizing and thinking of other things such as if the dogs ate, which hairstyle you need next and much more. This sex is boring and flat. Sex should be engaging and both parties, but you know, it cannot be 100 every time. And this is such a bad moment you can say, sex was bad.

When there is an injury

When you are busy having what is expected to be good sex, on the bed, car, or kitchen table, you may get injured. Your head may be hurt by utensils, he may bite your pussy or she may accidentally bite your dick (ouch). There and then, the pleasure will not be the same again, you will start nursing your injuries. It may seem funny now, bad that must have been in the category of bad sex. One lady told us of how the dude she was making out with bit her vagina, she screamed and pretended to be sick so that she could be out of there. Others have fallen out of the bed at the heat of the moment. I mean it's a long tale.

Sudden Fetish

Everyone has a desire and it is okay. However, it sounds different when it is sudden and unexpected. Like you are at the middle of sex and your partner whips your ass for him to cum. It can be crazy and scary if it was not communicated. This kind of sex falls under bad sex days.

Dry sex

It's horrible to have sex while there was zero for play. More so, when the lady is not wet. Most of the time the guy gets erect quickly and may not be aware that the girl needs to be ready too. But some will go on and start thrusting like a rabbit without concern. That results in horrible sex. Communicate as we discussed up there. Sex should be generous and not one lover being selfish.

Drunken

It's okay when it is consensual but you do not know what may happen to your partner. The side effects of drinking are worse. Your partner may throw up on you, another may snore while you are shagging and damn, isn't it bad. No one would love it.

Trial sex

You may decide to try new things that may end up going wrong. This may include using certain lubricants and one of you gets allergic to them. This does not go so well.

As we have noted, sex will not always be smooth, it will be meh sometimes. However, if you are in that relationship for the long term, there are solutions. Now, there is another issue of sexual compatibility. As you plan to revolve your sex life into a memorable mind-blowing moment, it is necessary to get an understanding of sexual compatibility. What is it, how do you tell if you are compatible? Let's find out.

Sexual Compatibility

There are many notions when it comes to the issue of compatibility. Most of the time while having our social chats, we term that people of the same caliber move together. This is to mean that partners with the same characteristics match. On the other hand, we are familiar with words such as the opposite characters attract. This means that finding a partner who has different characteristics than yours is your perfect match. Compatibility and similarity are closely related but not fully. Let's dive into demystifying what is compatibility. When we talk about partners being sexually compatible, it means that they feel that they are related in terms of preferences, sexual beliefs, sexual needs, and desires. The compatibility of partners is also measured to the rate in which individuals in a romantic relationship relate to the desires that turn them on and off emotionally, in terms of behavior, and cognitive.

Sexual compatibility among partners is closely related to satisfaction. Research shows that the more couples find themselves compatible, their sex life is revealed to be satisfying. On the other hand, sexual compatibility also develops the connection in a relationship. The more compatible one is, the better the relationship. In any case that any of the levels go down, the connection also goes down. This topic is not fully researched despite the finding that it helps in developing a thriving relationship. More research has continued to show that sexual compatibility is relevant in stabilizing sexual communication, the desire for sex, the act of sex, and communication. Sexual incompatibility stems from different likes and acts of inconsistency between partners regarding sex. When it comes to being turned on and off, there are instances such as one partner preferring sex with lights on while the other needs a dark environment, one may like it while drunk and the other while sober, one is turned on by fingering while the other is turned on by oral sex. Such instances may interfere with the compatibility of your relationship and the sexual satisfaction of each. This is because the desires of your partner are not fully met.

On the other hand, if you feel and think that you and your partner are compatible, it is a reflection your sex life will be satisfying. This will be in the assumption of the turning on and off of the stimulants of sexual desires. The general suggestion is that if you perceive you are compatible, then that is it. It is normal in our society to find partners all over loving each other, and then when something goes wrong they start throwing blame to each other. Personality compatibility also goes hand in hand with sexual compatibility. If you think that your personality type is compatible with your partner, then that is enough to say that your relationship can thrive. The instances where you have an argument and think you are not meant to be is vague. You stick to the perception because that's right. Therefore, even incompatibility, the instance you see your partner as a good match, one downside does not give you a green light to run away. You should give them another chance because you already have a good perception of each other. Research proofs that perception is right when it comes to sexual compatibility. While you blend with communication, then you can talk it out.

This is not to mean that some are not compatible, they are. Then if you do not perceive that you are a good match, the relationship will not have intimacy, and will in turn not lead to good satisfying sex life. In turn, the relationship might not work because you already do not perceive that you are compatible. In these instances, there will be no communication, because you cannot effectively communicate with your partner.

In this chapter, we can summarize that sexual intercourse is an important thing in a romantic relationship. Many ways stimulate your desire to have sex, that includes fingering, oral sex, and foreplay. It is also important that you communicate to your partner about sex and express your desires and fears. This will help in solving any problems that may be involved in the relationship. Therapy is a good place to seek help as well as counseling. You have also gotten that, coming out as a critique in sexual communication is dangerous for the relationship. The book has also further offered the benefits of having sex. There are numerous advantages that sex brings for both men and women. The book has highlighted instances that you may term sex as bad sex. It will not be always smooth and awesome. There are little awkward moments that will happen once in a while that will leave you feeling meh! Finally, the book has expounded on sexual compatibility. When you meet a partner, do not think that you will always feel compatible, but when you do, that is the best thing. Compatibility brings with it, emotional stability, effective ability to communicate, attraction, desires and a thriving relationship. With compatibility, there is a belief that you will be able to solve your relationship problems openly without judgment.

In the next chapter, we dive in to discuss the stimulants of sexual intercourse. Remember before you get into the mind bowing positions you need to be well aroused and that dick better is erect to do the did.

Chapter 2

Sexual stimulants

You have your desires and what turns you on or else arouses you have intercourse. That is your stimulant. As discussed in chapter one, every individual has their kind of fantasy and desire. Therefore, you cannot generalize that what turns your partner is what turns you. On the other hand, if you are not aware of what stimulates you to be wet or to have an erect dick, we got you. There are different kinds of stimulants.

Foreplay

Foreplay is all that happens before the intercourse. This includes touching, kissing, caressing, holding, dirty talking and much more. You should note that men become easily aroused visually, but as for women their needs some work. Women love the foreplay and would easily be turned off by a man who doesn't consider it, because what is the point of thrusting when you are not aroused to the moment. For women, foreplay is very important for them to be ready for penetrative sex. So how can you improve your foreplay? As long as your partner has consented to sex, there is no manual as to how you will perform the foreplay. Here are some examples that you can consider for your woman;

- Suck her nipples
- Kiss the back of her neck
- Caress her body smoothly
- Kiss her whole body the way she wants it
- Stroke her clitoris
- Fingering
- Tell her about all the good things you like about her
- Hold her tight and let your groin be felt

As for the men.

- Touch his testicles gently
- Stroke his penis
- Caress his body
- Lick that dick
- Lick his nipples
- Tell him he is sexy
- Kiss him passionately
- Touch him
- Tell him how you love sex with him
- Note his weak points and do what he desires

What does foreplay mean to men

A lot of men, if questioned do not think that foreplay is important. They do not consider to have had sex until the full penetrative action happens. The action means much more for them than the caressing. However, since we are talking about a man and a woman, then foreplay needs to happen because it means a lot for the lady. Just like in a menu, the woman may go for ice cream while the guy is interested in the meat. He is interested in getting his stomach packed, unlike the woman who is looking to feel good.

Fingering

At this point, you should note that stimulating arousal and desire for penetrative intercourse is very important. What is bad about having satisfaction when having intercourse is not about not doing something but rather initiating a great thing and flopping at it. This such thing is fingering. Research has shown that most men currently are doing nothing with fingering. Men, remember that fingering is not a measure of any fears that you may have. There is a potential of having a great fingering session with your woman if at all you will stop worrying and thinking of what you think are important things. A study has shown that men think other things are much more important than fingering. This includes the size of his dick. For crying out loud, a woman does not care whether you have a big or tiny dick when it comes to fingering. All she cares about is your fingers to do the thing. If you get it right, it will serve well if you have a small dick and it will be a bonus if your dick is the right size according to her. So, stop caring about your dick size and focus on giving her a fingering orgasm. Another thing that men have been found to focus on is giving her many orgasms. Orgasms are great, but can we enjoy the moment one step at a time. If you are at fingering, aim at giving her an organized orgasm from that act. The time that you will last is also a big concern. Psychologists' advice men that short mind-blowing sex is way better than long thrusting without much pleasure. Fingering is much better than that.

While fingering, getting to know the gist of it is necessary than not knowing what to do.

How to finger a girl

Prepare earlier Your preparation will include getting your hands clean. This is because the vagina is a very delicate organ that needs great care. Preparing through hygiene is a great way to avoid infection. Hands are exposed to different kinds of work, where you fetch bacteria and other infectious dirt.

Carry lubrication For a multitude of reasons, Lube is very essential. First, not all women, even in their high state of excitement, lubricate normally liberally. And for learners, if you neglected to switch it on correctly, it's secure to have a bottle of lubricant to relieve it with the finger movement. Finally, if you need to go all the way to the epic end, notice that some women later attain orgasm than others. By that moment, it may have drained out her natural juices, making a fast spritz of lube very useful.

Know her touch desires Ladies who caress themselves would realize the ideal recipe on arriving at a climax in the most pleasant manner they can. This is a significant hint to seeing how to finger a lady that a great many people ignore! Get access the best fingering counsel from the proprietor of the vagina. Notwithstanding that, this makes for a decent, prodding foreplay. Cuddle very close and request that her guide your turn in the correct places or request that that shrewd young lady "admit" how she contacts herself when she's considering you.

Be in a relaxed angle As referenced, young ladies set aside some effort to come to the "enormous O." If you're going for the panoramic detour of fingering moment, you should be in an agreeable situation to have the option to support the arousal until she cums. Sooner or later, your hands and arms tire out and moving position occasionally interferes with the incitement and vestiges the force.

Get her aroused Turning her on with foreplay before fingering is a valuable stunt to make the experience progressively pleasant for both. On the off chance that she's truly turned on, she greases up uninhibitedly and she reacts better to incitement. Also, obviously, who wouldn't appreciate seeing a horny, groaning lady powerless helpless before your fingers? when she is horny, you effectively do your thing till she gets an orgasm.

Sex talk Keeping correspondence open is a decent method to screen your development. This should be possible just by inquiring as to whether she's getting a charge out of what you're doing with your fingers. You could likewise incorporate grimy talk by disclosing that you like her reaction and that it arouses her desire more.

Focus on her expression The vast majority thinks that it's crazily good to watch a lady's response as she is fingered. Yet, besides this, watching her response tells if a specific development of your fingers is pleasurable or not. These aides you for which sort of fingering procedure you have to continue to have the option to carry her to a climax.

Know her life structures This implies realizing what sections of her body bring her pleasure when contacted and what sort of caress is appropriate for the different sections of her body. The parts include:

The clitoris the sacred goal of the entire pack, the clitoris is a little handle of tissue you find only underneath from the earliest starting point of the vulva cut. The clitoris is home to a large number of nerve receptors making it exceptionally touchy to contact. There are loads of approaches to invigorate the clitoris which evoke various reactions for each lady.

Vaginal canal This path of muscle is intended to suit a penis and permit the entry of an embryo during birth making it exceptionally touchy to inclusion weight. Human fingers then again, have lesser volume contrasted with a penis however being moveable makes for different incitement conceivable outcomes.

G-spot

The G-spot is a springy piece of the vagina situated on the foremost piece of the vagina or the upper part if the lady is resting down facing up. Whenever animated appropriately, it gives the most stunning all things considered. Anyway, there is no organized method to animate this, and it can fluctuate per individual.

Trial with various finger developments

As referenced, there are numerous approaches to finger a lady. Finding the correct kind of way to arouse her expects you to attempt different methods and developments to discover which one makes her groan more intense.

Use easy, brushing contacts-For the outside parts, for example, the clitoris and the labia. Light contacts to delicate zones is a decent method to turn her on and make her wet. Also, it gives her expectation making her responsive to forceful fingering later.

Make the action with your index and center finger-You need to begin with the center finger as it is the longest and has the more distant reach, particularly when invigorating the G-spot. Utilizing the two fingers is prescribed for G-spot incitement as it covers more surface zone than one finger alone.

Begin in slow motion and build up the thrust later-For you to learn how to finger her properly, you should slow down and be easy. Beginning in an easy motion allows her to get the flesh contact that also does wonders to her arousal. As you do it, focus on her expression. That way you will be aware of when to increase your speed and can also tell if she likes it.

Be touchy but don't touch the clitoris yet-the vagina and the clitoris are the sweet spots. The idea of avoiding them is to allow you to build the urge to penetrate, Avoid them at all cost to get maximum stimulation and arousal. When you do this, your partner will be craving for the penetration or the clit stimulation. Isn't it awesome when she demands it? Yes

Do multiple things as you finger-When you become a pro and touch the different sweet spots that arouse her, you will let her build an awesome orgasm. As you work with your fingers down there, let your lips be kissing her neck, as you whisper dirty words and suck her nipples. This will drive her nuts and satisfied.

Be still with the fingering

The mistake that you will make as a man is to stop fingering your woman before she comes. Some stop when the buildup of the orgasm is becoming intense. This can be awkward as she needs more time in the session to release her cum. That is the basic reason why you should focus on her expressions. When you note that she is almost at the climax, focus on the sweet spots until she cums.

ORAL SEX

Oral sex is a stimulant for arousal in an intimate relationship. It may feel different things to different people. If you like it, you can incorporate it into your relationship for great sex. Many terms are used to define oral sex such as blow job, giving head, or going down. Oral sex involves using your mouth to arouse your partner. Oral sex can be a decent method to find new delights with your accomplice, however choosing whether you need to do it is an extremely personal decision, not every person likes it and not every person attempts it! Likewise, with sex, it's significant that the two individuals are excited about doing it. We focus on the ways that you can have great oral sex with your partner.

To achieve the best oral sex

A great deal has been expounded on the most proficient method to give the best oral sex. In any case, various things work for various individuals.

There's an entire assortment of licking approaches, suck and invigorate. Various individuals may get a kick to give and get oral sex in various ways. Keep in mind that it can require a significant period to know what makes somebody feel better.

You may feel anxious before having oral sex regardless of whether you're giving it or accepting it. The best activity is to continue speaking with your accomplice. Request that they reveal to you what feels pleasant and let them know when you are appreciating something.

If you're glad and attracted to the individual, you're with, at that point oral sex can be an incredible method to get physically nearer and realize what turns each other on. Yet, recollect that you can respite or stop anytime you need, and the equivalent is valid for your accomplice. Because you have begun something doesn't mean you have to proceed – halting is in reality ordinary.

It is important to note that, oral sex for men and women is done differently. The basic reason is that the organs are not the same. Let us look at the ways to give oral sex to both men and women.

Men

While you are giving head to a man. It does not matter whether his dick is erect or not. It's a smart thought to utilize your hand to caress him before you begin to help work up to the impression of oral sex.

In case you're uncertain how far you need him to infiltrate your mouth, utilize your thumb and pointer to make a ring around his penis, halting it to the extent you need to go. You can hold moving your fingers down gradually until you arrive at the point where it feels profound enough in your mouth.

Numerous men discover oral sex exceptionally delicate, so start tenderly and gradually and work up to a quicker pace. You can explore different avenues regarding distinctive tongue, mouth and head developments to perceive what works best (however never utilize your teeth except if inquired!).

Regardless of whether you choose to give a man oral sex, it doesn't imply that you need to allow him to discharge/cum in your mouth, the final decision is yours. If he's wearing a condom this will be less problematic, and it implies are secured against explicitly transmitted diseases (STIs). It's additionally altogether up to you to what extent you proceed for.

Women

It's normally a smart thought to invest some energy kissing and contacting before giving a lady oral sex. Take as much time as necessary to go into her upper thighs and the territory around her vagina first, to enable her to get wet.

The most delicate piece of the vagina for a lady is the clitoris, which has more than 8,000 nerve endings. In any case, the entire pelvic zone is exceptionally touchy. Tenderly part the external lips of the vagina and search for the vaginal opening, and the hooded clitoris simply above it.

Start delicately, utilizing a casual tongue to make sluggish developments and work up to quicker developments with a firmer, pointed tongue. You can explore different avenues regarding making various examples with your tongue and attempt various rhythms – submitting general direction to your accomplice about what she appreciates most.

Oral anal sex

Oral anal sex is using your mouth to stimulate your partner through the anus. Performing oral sex on your accomplices rear-end (otherwise called analingus or rimming) can be a piece of any sexual relationship, regardless of whether gay, indiscriminate or straight.

If you are worried about cleanliness, request that your accomplice wash first water and a delicate washcloth ought to work. You could likewise wash together as a feature of foreplay.

You can start by delicately kissing and stroking the territory around the rear-end including the perineum (the region of skin between the privates and the butt). You would then be able to work your way into the butt by orbiting your tongue around the external region lastly embedding your tongue.

You can take a stab at licking, sucking, tasting and snacking tenderly – submitting general direction to your accomplice about what feels great to them.

On the off chance that you are performing it on a lady, don't go from the rear-end to the vagina as this may move microbes and cause contamination.

Is oral sex dangerous in any way?

There is a lower risk of getting infected with HIV through oral sex. The fundamental dangers emerge if the individual getting oral sex has an STI or bruises on their genital territory, or if the individual giving oral sex has injuries in their mouth or draining gums.

Anyway different STI for example, herpes, gonorrhea, and syphilis can, in any case, be gone on through oral sex. Furthermore, a few diseases brought about by microscopic organisms or infections can be gone on through oral–butt-centric sex, for example, hepatitis An or E.coli.

Contaminations can be gone on through oral sex regardless of whether there are no undeniable signs or side effects of the disease, (for example, bruises). You should abstain from having oral sex if both of you has injuries around your mouth, vagina, penis or butt. These could be an indication of a disease, so get them looked at by a medicinal services proficient.

Utilizing a condom or dental dam (a dainty, delicate plastic that covers the vagina or rear-ends) will shield you from most explicitly transmitted contaminations. If you don't have a dental dam, you can likewise make a successful obstruction by cutting a condom lengthways from base to top shaping one bit of material that can be utilized like a dental dam. Realizing you have the additional assurance a condom gives can help make you feel progressively freed and less repressed during oral sex. Conversing with your accomplice about security before you start having oral sex will enable things to go all the more easily. This can be humiliating, yet it's a significant piece of engaging in sexual relations and on the off chance that you discover it too hard to even think about discussing, at that point, it could be an indication that you aren't prepared to begin having oral sex presently.

In conclusion, It's a major choice to begin having oral sex, and, significantly, you and your accomplice are prepared to begin investigating thusly. Regardless of whether it's giving or accepting oral sex, nobody ought to do it since they feel compelled to. Lines as "it doesn't mean we've had genuine sex – regardless you'll be a virgin", or "on the off chance that you don't need sex, at that point you ought to in any event go down on me", or "it's not as hazardous as engaging in sexual relations", all propose weight and intimidation. Keep in mind that oral sex ought to be a good time for both of you. On the off chance that one individual is doing it since they feel constrained, it can sharp the entire experience.

Choosing whether to have oral sex is exceptionally close to the home thing. The primary interesting points are whether it feels right and whether you and your accomplice are both certain.

Eat her pussy like a pro

In opposition to what the vast majority think, ladies, fantasize on sex more than men do (they're simply better at concealing it.) Women long for a person who can give them a heart-beating, body-shaking climax. Ladies long for a person who knows precisely how to eat her pussy out... the correct way! Ladies are fixated on sex and are continually searching for a person who realizes how to eat her out until makes them dribble climax after the other. So my recommendation is to ensure you are that person so she doesn't look anyplace else. Do you need to give her a climax that 'keeps running up her spine' and makes her 'toes twist-up' simply considering it? At that point read these tips through and through. In all actuality, on the off chance that you don't think about these procedures, at that point, you hazard losing your lady to a person who knows them. I'm demonstrating how to eat a young lady with the goal that you nearly ensure she has a climax. Eating pussy is an artistic expression and it's something each person ought to figure out how to do or he hazards his young lady leaving him for a person who knows better. Most folks don't set aside the effort to contemplate female sexual joy. Although in this book I'm going to give you some incredible tips on the most proficient method to go down on her for the greatest climaxes in the least time.

Stimulate her

Getting your lady in the correct mood is one of the most essential parts of having the option to give her a climax. Ladies are enthusiastic animals, and it's difficult to give her a climax while she stays in a legitimate outlook (like when she's simply completed work or is worried.) This is the reason researchers consistently think that its difficult to ponder the female climax. It is your obligation and duty to get her loose, and turn her on with the goal that she disregards the anxieties and stresses of life – this is the thing that foreplay is about. What's more, not normal for men, ladies take any longer to get in the state of mind. Perhaps you can prepare an erection and get for sex inside 10 seconds, for ladies it could take thirty minutes or more. This is the point at which the sexual vitality and excitement develop.

Create anxiety

Prodding and foreplay is the place the intensity of the climax originates from. Envision you have an enormous container at the highest point of a stepping stool. The container holds water, however first you have to top off the can with water. Your point with the pail is to make the greatest and most emotional blast conceivable when you, at last, choose to push the basin of water off the stepping stool. You could simply place a smidgen of water in the basin and after that drive it off. Be that as it may, the blast of water wouldn't be extremely enormous. You could invest more energy topping off the container and when you, at last, pushed the basin off the stepping stool the blast was colossal. The water resembles female sexual vitality. It needs time and foreplay to develop, yet the more you take to develop her vitality, the greater the climax blast will be toward the end. I've composed a total guide about how to make a lady wet appropriate here.

Cover her eyes

Probably the most ideal approaches to expand expectation and excitement is to utilize props. Since ladies can likewise be reluctant about sex, and particularly about when they get their vagina licked out, a blindfold can be an incredible method to make her vibe less hesitant, and rather simply appreciate the sensations. Utilizing a blindfold on her likewise has the additional impact of lessening one of her detects. At the point when her sight is turned off her impression of touch will enormously increment. She will feel the sensations and incitement from her pussy quite a lot more. It's additionally marginally alarming wearing a blindfold. You will have unlimited oversight over her (which ladies love) and her feeling of fervor and expectation will increment.

There are many ways to eat pussy. This includes sucking, blowing, kissing and licking.

Blowing

Blowing on her pussy is an extraordinary type of excitement, foreplay, and prodding. The light, unpretentious sensation will start to make sexual vitality and pressure (which gets discharged in a climax)

The blowing is light, it prods and stimulates her. It draws her consideration and spotlight on to the inconspicuous sensations she feels in her pussy.

This is actually what you need. You need her in a condition of extreme touchiness. Each never in her vagina will begin shivering with sensations.

Licking is straightaway. You would now be able to begin to utilize your tongue in light movements over her delicate parts.

It's essential to make your developments light and eccentric, to begin with. Despite everything, you need to prod her. Regardless you need her to hold up in expectation (as her sexual vitality keeps on the structure.)

Keep her speculating about when and how you will lick her next.

As her degree of sexual excitement keeps on rising, presently you can start to truly begin licking her out (and above all her clit)

The here and there movement, delicately over her clit is typically the best choice.

You ought to change your strokes. From moderate and delicate to quick and hard. Continuously search for her responses so you can see or hear what she prefers best.

Kissing

Kissing her cooch is an extraordinary method to indicate the amount you care about her. You shouldn't kiss her vagina for a long time however, yet your kissing ought to be blended in with different strategies.

Sucking

Sucking is the following phase of delight and most ladies LOVE having their vagina sucked. Presently you can begin utilizing your entire mouth to animate her clit, however the remainder of her vagina as well.

As her excitement levels move increasingly elevated she'll before long be prepared for climax however you should keep constructing to an ever-increasing extent.

Increment the speed and power of the sucking.

Continuously make sure to prod and go two stages forward, one stage back. Suck on her female bits for some time, at that point venture back and kiss, lick and blow before continuing.

Motorboating and Humming
This is the final technique that you'll utilize. It is maybe the most dominant. *Here's the way to do it...*

Put your lips delicately on her vagina. Let your lips simply daintily contacting and after that victory with the goal that your lips vibrate to and fro. It sends vibrations down through her pussy. These demonstrations like shockwaves that can trigger a climax to occur. Numerous ladies guarantee this is one of their preferred sensations. You can change the speed, power, and recurrence of the vibrations by holding your lips more tightly or blowing harder. Do not to go insane, however. With the motorboating strategy, you'll need to hold your lips over her clit and the opening to her vagina even though you can move it around and see where gives the best incitement. Murmuring is like motorboating yet rather than giving your lips a chance to move your essentially lean your mouth against her vagina and hmmm delicately. This sends vibrations straightforwardly into her pussy that is incredibly pleasurable. For the best outcomes, go to and fro between the techniques. Blend it up and keep her speculating. In any case, when you feel like she is exceptionally near the climax, at that point adhere to the technique that got her there and don't transform it to an extreme.

Sex toys

Sex toys are stimulants for both men and women. This is especially in a woman who needs her clit stimulated to the maximal, to be aroused. Couples can bring in different types of toys for different functions in the bedroom. Someplace along the line, an awful number of men have built up the worry that carrying toys into the room means they're explicitly insufficient here and there. Try not to be one of them! Most of the ladies need clitoral incitement (instead of just entrance) to climax—so except if you have a go-go device penis, penetrative sex alone won't get a lady off (however, truly, despite everything she enjoys it). Adding a vibrator to the blend demonstrates you know how the female body functions, and that you care about the amount she appreciates the merriments. It likewise lets her know you're explicitly brave. These are altogether alluring characteristics in a sex-have. The end product to men keeping away from sex toys is that dicks are significantly underserved with regards to determination. Hence, the vast majority of these models have clitorises as a top priority. On the in addition to side, there's a wide assortment from vibrators that twofold as the top of the line adornments to couples' toys to prostate pleasures, we've discovered verified picks for giving everybody included the endowment of climax.

Why should you use sex toys

Toys spice up the sex game.

When you decide to use sex toys, it varies if your partner is involved or not. If your a single woman, at that point sex toys are incredible approaches to study your body and simply become increasingly OK with your very own sexuality. For women, you get the opportunity to realize what you like, how you like, what are the catches that you have to push to pick up the most serious climaxes. Indeed, you can accomplish things with fingers, yet sex toys are structured by science. Vibrators are made to create the most extraordinary vibrations. G-spot dildos are intended to easily push on the G-spot for an opportunity to accomplish vaginal and clitoral climax, or notwithstanding squirting climax at the equivalent time. Since these pocket pussies are so great, they will recreate the genuine fervor that sex would give. An extraordinary method to prepare continuance. For couples, I'm certain you realize that least demanding approach to include energy and revive connections is simply to change area by traveling. Yet, that is not constantly conceivable. What are your alternatives at that point? : you can read books for new positions, stunts and pretends to attempt or... you just purchase another sort of sex toy and trial with that. If you believe that the trio is energizing... Then this is comparable. You're including an additional toy that you utilize together. It's new, it's energizing.

You get to the climax fast

It requires a lot of exertion for instance for you as a man to get her to the mood through her clit and lick the pussy simply the correct way.

The tongue gets drained brisk. At the point where I am stimulating her g-spot, you become tired and drained quick and my continuance is what's preventing her from arriving at an amazing vaginal or squirting climax. At last, there is coordination. If you need to include butt-centric incitement, you have to stress over cleanliness. With a butt plug, for instance, all the experience just ends up simpler and progressively pleasurable. Indeed, even as you stroke off without anyone else's input you have to work less and you can concentrate more on your body feeling the delights. Imagine a scenario in which you need butt-centric incitement, clitoral, vaginal... and bosom incitement simultaneously. It is impractical in an ordinary event. Be that as it may, attempt the hare vibrator and you will get vaginal and clitoral incitement by utilizing one hand... and you have a free second hand to do whatever you like!

They bring a new feeling that you could not experience without

Indeed, there is a particular sort of sensations you get by utilizing your fingers while stroking off.

There are various sensations when you are engaging in sexual relations with your accomplice.

Sex toys add additional shades to sexual play.

For instance, with a rooster ring on fellow's penis, you can all of a sudden encounter a greater, firm and full penis. With a tie on, you could peg your accomplice. A prostate massage can help your man get arousal faster with minimal exertion. You can experience the great orgasm when stimulated with fingers, a butt plug, or a dildo. This can also be effective if you are trying to achieve a great anal orgasm. At that point there are all the fun couples play toys like remote control vibrators that you can use in broad daylight to mess around with. Truly, and if you like the additional filling background you could attempt mythical serpent size dildos even horse dildos. The last model there are additionally penis sleeves that your person could put over his penis if he's littler than normal.

Sex toys can immensely improve your intimacy by giving you a new kind of orgasm

On the off chance that you've seen the grown-up motion pictures and have seen ladies having full-body climaxes with squirting. What's more, you've pondered is this conceivable? Or then again you've seen folks talk about non-ejaculatory different climaxes through prostate draining. Also, pondered is it genuine? Sex toys can enable you to find these sort of incredible climaxes quicker and simpler. Truly, it's conceivable to accomplish the majority of this without sex toys. Be that as it may, the sexual well-being industry is creating. there is a site which spotlights on understanding the science behind ladies' pleasure and disclosing how to hit the correct spots, how to set up the body for progressively exceptional climaxes. What's more, indeed, it's generally finished with the assistance of sex toys. It's a billion-dollar industry and organizations are buckling down on making the best joy gadgets. Presently, the new pattern is the keen sex toys that help you comprehend your climaxes so every next one show signs of improvement's and better. Some vibrators can assist you to reach your orgasm and also discover numerous ways that you were not aware of. These vibrators include the g-spot mental wand.

There are different toys for different functions for both men and women. Let's have a look.

Vibrators

Various examinations have demonstrated that around 80% of ladies don't climax from intercourse. Truly, they need clitoral incitement. Along these lines, it's just clear that vibrators are the primary thing we center around that is the top ladies delight toy.

The magic wand massager

This is the most popular vibrator that began the vibrator ladies joy sex toy industry. You can't turn out badly with this one.

It accompanies two amazing velocities and truly, you can utilize it to back rub out your sore back and whatever else. The extraordinary thing about Hitachi is that you can purchase numerous connections over it — like hare vibrator connection and vacillate wand connection (attempt it!!) This model will last you for a considerable length of time!

Dildos

Dildos are incredible on the off chance that you don't have an accomplice or you essentially appreciate the filling sentiment of dildo. You can go as sensible as you need or as insane as you need. A few ladies love gigantic dildos that give filling sensations. A few ladies love dream type dildos like — monster, horse, hound, limb dildos.

Bunny vibrators

Those are toys 2 out of 1. A definitive sex toy as I would see it.

You can get pushing, pivoting or vibrating dildo + vibrator over it...!

Butt plugs

OK, presently we're entering the butt-centric play. Butt fittings are an incredible expansion to any couples play or solo play. What you do is you essentially embed the lubed butt plug... and that is it!!! What you get is new extraordinary sort of filling sensations. I recollect when I even had a go at placing just finger in my young ladies butt while screwing here — both I and she came capably before long! There was only something in the unusual, the totality of that additional little touch. You can just put the butt plugin and go on with ordinary sex... and it will be unique.

Or then again you can utilize them as butt-centric preparing to get ready for something greater in there.

For Men

There are two major sex toys each man should attempt:
Flesh light-the fake reproduction of lady's vagina (blended with Flashlight Launch screwing machine it makes a touchy combo)
Prostate Massager-truth is, men have significantly a larger number of motivations to attempt butt-centric play than ladies since they have P-detect, the male G-spot covered up there!

Flashlights are exceptional and serious.
As it goes to prostate massager, prostate draining is it's very own gigantic theme.
Indeed, men can accomplish prostate climax utilizing only their fingers, however utilizing a massager will make it so a lot simpler. You'll have the option to concentrate on the joy, not on the coordination of the procedure.

Here's how prostate climax feels like:
OK, we're in for the last stretch... !

The couples sex toys!

Contingent upon what you like or need these sex toys will spice up your sexual desire. What's more, obviously you can generally blend the recently referenced sex toys in there as well.

Remote Control Vibrators

Individuals regularly look for vibrating undies as they've heard they can be a fun remote open understanding.

Be that as it may, what they are searching for are egg vibrators which have a remote control. The issue with undies is that they don't hold in the spot. Be that as it may, with an insertable vibrator, you can't go wrong! It costs more, yet this is because most less expensive toys experience difficulty with range, network, and clamor.

Love sense

Love sense vibrator is uncommonly bent to touch the G-spot and the battery keep going for as long as 4 hours with 7 vibration modes. It has an incredible Bluetooth association you can control the gadget using your telephone.

The telephone is very attentive and you can see the intensity of vibrations in plain view constantly. It works either in 30–45 feet go on the off chance that you use Bluetooth association. Be that as it may, it works any separation if you control it through the Internet.

No doubt... this implies you could request that she put it in and bother her regardless of whether she's not there. She can at present turn it off if you don't hit the ideal time, yet you can screen everything on the telephone.

Strap ons

It is safe to say that you are keen on pegging background?

Better believe it, you could purchase an outfit a unique dildo and screw your male accomplice (or female accomplice in case you're lesbian) in the butt...!

That is unusual, in certainty it was my sweetheart's #1 dream..! ;) You can purchase saddle and dildos independently.

Or on the other hand, you can purchase strapless tie on dildo where one end is embedded in lady's vagina so she gets a physical joy while she's pushing as well.

Rooster Rings

A few people love the way chicken rings look and use them in unusual BDSM play. Some folks have erection issues and they use penis siphons to get erect. A short time later they put on a rooster ring to counteract for blood to leave the penis. Along these lines, they can appreciate ordinary sex for around 20 minutes notwithstanding their inabilities.

Be that as it may, most couples use cockerel rings to get very hard, greater than normal size and circumference penis. It's 100% safe to use for around 20 minutes... and huge amounts of fun!

Penis sleeves

They are essentially penis expansions and generally, folks use them on the off chance that they are little estimated. This is an extraordinary method to cheat, give their spouses an energizing greater delight while inclining that they are the ones doing the screwing. Envision penis sleeves like extremely thick condoms... :)

Sex Swings

At long last, in case you're looking a fun method to appreciate weightless sex understanding and have pleasant cardio simultaneously... sex swings may be the perfect thing for you!

The main cautioning is that they either take a great deal of room or will require penetrating unique snares in the roof.

Be that as it may, you can generally conceal them with the hanging plants!

The entryway swings are anything but difficult to introduce, however they are not so much agreeable and entryways may not hold.

You can generally lie and state that you're rehearsing yoga there and have a ton of fun simultaneously!

Prostate incitement can be supernatural, similar to you don't know where the delight is coming from. Penis incitement, presently, while still decent, is more to the point. Very surprising. Prostate incitement feels blunter and less extreme in the feeling of concentrated fervor, however exceptionally incredible and serious in an all the more full-body experience way.

Chapter 3

Sex Positions

Introduction to sex positions

Let me begin by asking you if you had sex positions in your yearly goals. I mean if you are in an intimate relationship, this should be one of the goals. If not, its never too late. This book is going to show you the various positions that you will try in your intimate moments. You do not have to stick to one position making it normal and boring.

Importance of sex positions

You get a different view

During the change of positions, you also get to change the places of accomplices as to one another, accordingly, you change viewpoints, perspectives and snugness of accomplices' bodies. As such: You change the image they see. Also, in its turn, the image impacts the accomplices' view of what is happening and their sentiments. It is particularly significant for men, as their eyes are the subsequent delicate zone after penis on its significance. It does not shock anyone that ladies love with their ears and men with their eyes!)) Men to a great extent live the sex outwardly, that is the reason they cherish such a great amount to watch pornography. Hearing, the feeling of touch and smell of men are additionally initiated during sex, however, above all, they are energized by the image, that is the thing that they see. For instance, when a man and a lady do it in the missionary position when the couple can see only the essences of one another. Furthermore, for instance, doggy style places of the opened female rider, when the man see a brilliant perspective on lady's rump and when he sees his penis infiltrate into his female accomplice and makes her shudder of joy. You should concede that just from the visual side these two positions will wakeful completely various feelings of the man and in doggy style positions his feelings will be a lot more brilliant. All things considered, men will comprehend what we are discussing!) With a difference for men, for ladies the most significant discernment channels after genitals are skin and ears. That is the reason they cherish so a lot of delicate words and long-term delicate caresses, kiss, and strokes on the body.

It brings different expressions

To see better the interconnection between all sex positions as well as the sentiments you got that you have to comprehend the accompanying things: in each position the penis enters under various point and with various profundity by invigorating various pieces of the vagina, its various zones and with various force. As the inward surface of the vagina is sullied (has diverse reasonableness), the sentiment of a lady in various positions will be additionally extraordinary. At that, each lady has her sentiments, which can contrast from the sentiment of another lady. Men, in this connection, have nearly a similar circumstance: in various positions, they have a diverse effect on the leader of their penis, on its various territories. That implies that:

Various situations for sex permit changing force of incitement and zones of incitement of the vagina by the penis. Furthermore, as these zones have distinctive reasonableness, the couple can encounter various emotions.

Arousal of Various feelings
Another view, different sentiments and different feelings. Past variables are taken together brought into the world the third factor. Attempting differentiated positions, you soak your adoration game with various hues and shades that are with various feelings. We have just discussed the significance of assorted variety in sex to save enthusiasm. Various positions are probably the least complex approaches to accomplish it.

Replacement for incompatibility

We as a whole know the situations when the man has a smaller penis and the lady cannot get delighted. On the other hand, when the man has a too huge penis, which makes the lady experience more disagreeable sentiments than wonderful. Be that as it may, luckily, such inconsistency can be effectively disposed of with the assistance of exceptional sex positions. Different sex positions will help your partner stroke and meet the sexual desires of the other partner. for example, where missionary style cannot help, doggy style may serve.

Arousal of different sweet spots

In the purpose of reality, that is the thing that we have just examined in the area "Various emotions", yet here we might want to stress one significant truth. We're talking around 3 primary sexy zones of the vagina. When you think about their reality and their exact area in the vagina, you can deliberately animate them, passing on various types of the climax of the lady. See, when you have different sex positions, the sweet spots will be hit differently, therefore, making the sex sweeter since it is satisfying.

Give the lady what she needs from the climax.

Each lady and her sexuality is a special book which you should get it. In contrast to the lady, the man can get climax in completely every sex position, as in any position his penis head is animated enough well. Also, if we talk about the lady, at that point, it is increasingly troublesome. The lady's clitoris on its size, position, and reasonableness contrast among various ladies, as they have the distinctive culmination of touchy focuses on their vaginas, which we referenced previously.

Every one of that prompts the way that on the off chance that you need to fulfill the young lady normally you have to see how to more readily animate and to give them more consideration during sex. How might you decide all that? – You have to analyze to an ever-increasing extent! It is amazing, yet much of the time, the young ladies comprehend what they should be fulfilled, how and where to invigorate, at what profundity and with what force. Directly for that, there exist a lot of sex positions which can enable you to invigorate the lady in various ways, and finely you will comprehend what she enjoys the greater part of all.

Conditioning the entire living being

In the oriental prescription there exists such a thought as reflection. It is about the reality, that all pieces of body and all organs of our living being are associated and by impacting on one organ in some exceptional manner you can in a roundabout way effect on others. Privates are not an exemption. Both man's penis and lady's vagina from inside on their surface have numerous agent regions of every single crucial organ that are focuses which are associated with these organs. That is the reason, the more genital regions you invigorate during sex, the bigger conditioning impact to the entire life-form of the two accomplices will be.

Now let us look at the different sex positions that types of sex positions.

Sex positions that will help you connect with your partner

Sex is regarded as the most brilliant and private exercises that you and your life partner can share. It improves your connection, builds your longing for one another, advances great well-being and the offers the capacity to grasp calls of wants from your companion which are on the whole endowments from God.

On the off chance that you just became a couple and have a desire to connect more intimately, on the off chance that you have been hitched for some time and need a few situations to reconnect with your life partner, we have curated the 10 best sex positions for you to do as such! Keep reading.

The Missionary position

Alright, so this probably won't be anything new, yet the great missionary isn't exemplary for reasons unknown! This is a rundown of the "best sex positions to associate with your life partner" all things considered, and there's nothing progressively cozy, not all that much, nothing more consoling than sexual closeness preacher style which is the reason it makes it to the top spot in our 10 best sex positions.

In this position, the lady relaxes on her back with her legs laying level on the bed. The spouse enters her while in this position. There is a chance of enhancing this position, by putting a little pad under the lady's bum to raise her a little bit higher. This wind offers further entrance, which is useful for when you are attempting to get a baby. Still in this position, the woman can wrap her legs around the hips of her man, this gives him a chance to do some direct strokes, and the woman feels the penis go deep, hence bring her satisfaction. The missionary position is very comfortable to couples and it is a go-to position when you feel tired of the intense positions. It gives you a chance to face your partner's eyes and feel the connection. Nothing greater than that.

Spooning

After a busy day of work for both of you, you can both appreciate the loosening up way that spooning gives you a chance to get physically involved with your life partner. It enables men to unwind, yet at the same time gives them full access to their lady. This position is very simple. This is how it is done. You are both lying on the bed, the guy behind the lady, and basically enters her pussy from behind. As simple as that.

The cowgirl position

Study shows that women love this position. This is a style whereby, the woman is on top. She is in control of doing her thing. This position has been found to give women multiple and intense orgasms. While on top she can see the expression of her partner and move with the pace until both of them reach the climax. How do you do this position? The guy lies down and the woman is on top. Period.

The cuddle squat

With this position, the guy sits facing his partner. The woman is sitting on her mans erection and thrusts up and down, while the guy holds her tight. It is the best position to cuddle, get satisfied and have an orgasm.

69 position

The 69 position has both of you facing different sides. In essence, the woman will be facing the guy's genitals and the same to the man. You can suck the dick as he licks the pussy. This position needs utmost vulnerability to let yourself loose to your partner. This positions scream that you want each other, and brings the best sensation for oral sex.

The Kneel position

This position needs you and your spouse kneeling facing each other. You are free to touch and caress as you enter and have intercourse.

Koala position

In this one, the husband carries the wife. This will be a little difficult in terms of weight. But, we strive to try new positions.

As the husband carries the wife, he holds her buts as he thrusts in. Enjoy!

We have looked at the positions that you should be trying as a couple. Now let us go forward and see some of the not so new styles that you can try this year.

Positions that will help you reach your climax

The cat position

Why it is awesome This contorts on missionary position develops intense clitoral incitement for your lover, a study has discovered that ladies who experienced difficulty arriving at a climax during the missionary style were bound to climax utilizing the coital arrangement style. How to attempt it: Start in with the famous missionary style and move your body up and over to the other side. Shake forward and back as opposed to pushing here and there to enable you to keep in touch with her clitoris.

Chair position

Why it's wonderful: If you have not aced standing positions, slip onto them with this one. It will give serious and profound entrance to her. Step by step instructions to attempt it: Lean your luck run out as if you're doing a divider sit. Your legs ought to be bowed nearly to a correct point and close enough together that she can straddle you.

You may find that it takes more time to focus to keep your equalization, your hands are allowed to lay on her hips, play with her bosoms, or stroke her back as you push. Contingent upon her stature, her feet probably won't have the option to contact the floor. On the off chance that it gets excessively tiring, structure a tripod by having her drop one of her feet to the floor, which makes it simpler on your legs.

Maypole position

Why it's great: it's a bit crazy, and the task can feel very exciting. Plus, her clitoris will squeeze toward your pelvic bone, rendering it more pleasing to her. How to attempt it: Have her wrap her legs around you starting from the place of the chair. Then, let her lay back and pick her up with your palms under her butt and move to a nearly upright place. Lift your shaft up and down. Keep your knees mildly twisted to assist hold your power.

Twist and shout position

Why it's amazing: This sex style is moderate and empowers further deep intercourse. It's likewise too personal since you're ready to see her body while keeping in touch. Step by step instructions to attempt it: Lie on your back as though you're prepared to do a sit-up, however with one leg reached out and the other twisted. Have her straddle one of your legs. She would then be able to go all over your penis, controlling the profundity and speed. Contingent upon which side your penis normally bends, she can sit and pound against you the other way of the bend, which should feel incredible for you.

Cowgirl cradled

Why it's wonderful: This position is extraordinary when you need to give her clitoral incitement, while as yet keeping up the closeness and closeness that some other eyes to eye positions bring. Instructions to attempt it: Instead of expecting the conventional sitting-up cowgirl position, have her lay forward with the goal that her face is supported into your neck. This can help adjust your bodies to give more straightforward clitoral incitement. You have your hands allowed to hold her hips, or for included delight, you can stretch around and invigorate her butt, if she's into that.

Backdoor Oral

Why it's amazing: "This can be an unexpected sensation in comparison to normal oral sex positions, as you are coming at it from behind instead of in front," says Wood.

Step by step instructions to attempt it: Have her lay on her stomach and spot a pad under her hips, which will help lift her butt so you have simpler access to her vulva, says Wood. This likewise leaves your hands allowed to embed a finger or two into her vagina for some inside incitement simultaneously.

Doggy style

Why it's marvelous: It's an incredible turn on the exemplary doggy style position, however, it doesn't require as much quality or adaptability from both of you, as stated by an authorized marriage specialist and creator of Classic Positions Reinvented. Furthermore, from this edge, it's somewhat simpler for you or her to physically animate her clitoris.

The most effective method to attempt it: Have her lay face down with her butt brought up noticeable all around for simple access. Your legs ought to be near one another inside hers. For more help, she can put a cushion under her stomach or prop herself up with her lower arms with her hands encircling her head and neck. To make it increasingly serious, place your hands on her back or hips so you can push with more power.

Double Decker style

Why it's wonderful: This is a simple change from any lady on-top position. Also, this edge gives you a chance to see her body respond to your pushing and your hands are allowed to wander her entire body from her bosoms right down to her clitoris.

The most effective method to attempt it: Start backward cowgirl. Have her recline until she's propped on her elbows, with her back on your chest and her arms supporting her body weight. Hold her at her abdomen to keep up more authority over the musicality of your pushing.

Galley Style

Why it's great: Watching her assume responsibility can be a rush. Also, if she's into butt-centric play, you can utilize your fingers from this position. This additionally offers her a chance to utilize a sex toy on her clitoris. (This vibrator has four distinctive power levels and vibration designs, so you can modify it to her needs.)

Step by step instructions to attempt it: This is a variety of switch cowgirl. Sit with your legs forward and recline on your arms. She will rest on your legs with her head close to your feet and straddle you at the hips, utilizing her arms for help. Her legs ought to be loosened up behind her, yet can be twisted at the knees for more help. You can put your hands on her butt and drive her to and fro here.

Twisted spoon

Why it's wonderful: This spooning variety gives profound infiltration yet isn't physically burdening like doggy style, as researched by a human sexuality researcher. Besides, it makes progressively pressure in both of your bodies, which effectively amps up excitement, she says.

Step by step instructions to attempt it: Both of you will lie on your sides, with you behind her. Have her raise her top leg noticeable all around. She should clutch her raised leg's lower leg while you push from behind. To truly make her go, invigorate her bosoms or clitoris or have her utilization a sex toy while you push.

Duet style

Why it's great: "Masturbation is perhaps the most ideal approaches to become acquainted with your own body, how you experience joy, and at last how an accomplice can fulfill you. This is a most optimized plan of attack to instructing your accomplice what works best for you and feels incredible simultaneously," says Amie Harwick, Ph.D., M.F.T., a California-based marriage and family advisor and creator of The New Sex Bible for Women.

Besides, you'll get the chance to see precisely how she gets a kick out of the chance to be contacted, as well. What's more, the perspective on her doing it isn't awful.

Step by step instructions to attempt it: Ask your accomplice to contact herself while you caress yourself. She may be bashful from the outset. If that is the situation, have her protest in front of you and lean her once again into your chest to make it increasingly agreeable and less intrusive inclination.

You can begin by contacting her body as she strokes off and steps by step start contacting yourself, so you both wind up participating in masturbation.

ORGASM

A climax is an outward reflex that happens when the muscles fix during sexual excitement and after that unwind through a progression of cadenced compression. Each peak can feel diverse regarding force and span, contingent upon how and what some portion of your body is being excited. Other than giving a physical discharge, it's additionally an enthusiastic one enabling you to feel nearer to your accomplice or essentially de-worry following an extreme day.

A few sorts of orgasm center around the vagina in particular; others enable you to feel the earth-convulsing force in spots you never thought of as erogenous zones. You deserve to discover the delight your body can understanding—enable us to get you up to speed with all the distinctive Os out there. Any sort of climax feels staggering, and there's nothing amiss with adhering to the strokes and contacts that you know carry you to the edge without fail. In any the same old thing, all the time wears out a person's soul. You wouldn't eat a similar three suppers consistently, nor would you wear a similar outfit again and again.

Types of orgasm

Clitoral climax

For most ladies, the clitoris is the all-around sweet spot when they need to encounter the joy and arrival of a climax. In any case, while clitoral climaxes might be the most available kind, this little, for the most part, shrouded joy catch is profoundly individualistic. Each lady favors an alternate kind of touch here to arrive at the peak.

The clitoris is an extremely delicate piece of a lady's life structures, made out of multiple nerves endings like that of the penis. Having it contacted, touched, or stroked using immediate or backhanded incitement (at the end of the day, through texture, or by contacting the labia encompassing the clitoris) prompts an expansion in the bloodstream to the territory, making the clitoris engorged and needing discharge.

An examination found that few kinds of clitoral strokes (brainstorm and-down, to and fro, and both wide and little circles) can prompt climax. Examination all alone and demonstrate your accomplice what you like. On the off chance that clitoral climaxes don't come simply for you or you are experiencing difficulty arriving at the peak, consider investigating sex toys structured in light of clitoral climax, for example, a smaller than usual vibrator you or your accomplice can wear on your fingertips.

G-spot climax

Your G-spot is on the front mass of your vagina, somewhere between your vaginal opening and cervix. It's not something you can see but rather you can, for the most part, feel it; embed a finger into your vagina and press forward (making a come-here movement). You ought to recognize a somewhat uneven or furrowed region. For certain ladies, it feels springy.

Squeezing this spot delicately and stroking it softly is the thing that numerous ladies do to prime themselves for a G-spot climax, otherwise called a vaginal climax. When you're explicitly stirred, the G-spot will top with blood and swell off. Contacting it such that feels great to you with fingers, your accomplice's penis, or a vibrator can trigger what numerous ladies portray as a profoundly extraordinary, deeply shaken sort of peak.

Mixed climax

If you can deal with two, three, or even multiple times the power and delight of a normal O, this sort of climax is for you. A mixed climax is a peak that happens when more than one erogenous zone is being aroused simultaneously. G-spot infiltration alongside clitoral contacting is one approach to encounter the dangerous climax that ordinarily results. In any case, it could likewise originate from vaginal entrance alongside clitoral, areola, or butt-centric incitement—or these at the same time.

The more incitement there is, the more bloodstream will result, and the greater the result of the climax. Numerous mixes of contacting and prodding can trigger a mixed climax, yet in case you're hoping to have one with an accomplice, think about the lady on top position (your hands, and your partner's, are allowed to contact your clitoris, bosoms, or butt) or carrying a vibrator into the room.

Anal climax

Butt-centric sex or butt-centric play isn't interesting to everyone. Some adoration it and others couldn't care less for it by any means. However, in case you're in the previous class (or you've never attempted it and figure you maybe), a butt-centric climax is one you should think about.

Since the anus and rectum are close to the clitoris and the vagina, they are associated by perineum which is a meager stretch of tissue where they share a large number of similar nerves and muscles, which include the PC pelvic floor of the muscle. The PC muscle is profoundly touchy for some ladies, and invigorating it can trigger a vaginal climax and also for the butt-centric.

If you are not sure about anal sex, you can look at the review from the numerous ladies who do report having climaxes from butt-centric sex. In any case, this kind of sex comes with dangers that are imperative to consider before you attempt it. Safe sex is an unquestionable requirement for you and your accomplice.

Profound vaginal erogenous zone climax

The clitoris and G-spot aren't the main joy catches unsportsmanlike. Genuine ladies just as sex analysts state that there are extra erogenous zones inside the vagina that when contacted the correct way can prompt what's all in all known as a profound vaginal climax.

First comes the A-spot, situated on the high front (or foremost) mass of the vagina just underneath the cervix. Next is the O-spot (for the climax), which can be found on the back mass of the vagina, practically behind the cervix. The tendons here contain nerves that give off an impression of being exceptionally delicate for some ladies. If fingers, a toy, or a penis fills the vagina enough at the high part of the bargain those nerves are truly invigorated, it tends to be extremely, pleasurable. It could make the entire uterus contract during a climax—there can be monstrous compressions in the entire region.

Squirting climax

Indeed, female discharge truly exists; it's the sign of this sort of climax. At times when ladies are explicitly excited or invigorated there is an ejection of liquid from the organs around the urethra or front surface of the vagina during or before the climax. However, it's still fervently challenged where the liquid originates from. The liquid is regularly clear and doesn't take after pee, and there can be a moderate sum discharged or an all-out spout.

G-spot incitement is the kind of contacting that regularly prompts squirting. Yet, stroking and prodding the zone encompassing the urethra has likewise been known to bring about a splash the-sheets peak. Nobody truly knows the precise number of ladies who experience a squirting climax, so in light of that vulnerability, it was discovered that 10-half of ladies have, at once or another, had a 'spouting' minute during the climax.

Cervical climax

You may just think about your cervix as far as a pelvic test or pregnancy, however, it very well may be a noteworthy erogenous zone too and produce its one of a kind sort of climax, says Dr. Lobby. It's not something each lady will understand since the cervix can likewise be too delicate to even think about directing touch. In any case, cervical incitement is connected to solid, exceptional climaxes, she says. It's ideal to attempt a cervical climax when you're very stirred and have had heaps of foreplay, which can make your cervix increasingly open to contact. Have a go at having your accomplice utilize moderate, profound strokes, or if his penis is excessively, use fingers or a vibrator. Simply don't drive it if it's not working for you there are a lot of different approaches to encounter an O.

The Nipple Orgasm

You know your bosoms and areolas are major erogenous zones; your areolas particularly respond to being contacted and stroked, since they're stacked with nerve endings and very delicate skin. In any case, a few ladies truly can encounter a major O just by having their areolas touched and kissed. There's no reasonable agreement on what number of ladies can climax with no cowardly contact, and scientists aren't sure why areola climaxes occur. Yet, if the thought interests to you, you could have a great deal of fun attempting to make sense of it. With enough kissing, sucking, and touching, these are zones that can carry some lady to climax.

Exercise climax

Arriving at peak while occupied with an extreme exercise may sound somewhat peculiar. Yet, exercise actuated climaxes, or orgasms, are genuine. An investigation revealed that over 300 ladies out of the 600 reviewed had encountered climax or sexual delight while working out, as a rule from center-based activities.

"One of the approaches to incite a climax is to super-crush your PC muscles and you can create them and make them more grounded. On the off chance that somebody has very much created PC muscles and during activities, they truly begin to contract them, I think climaxes are conceivable during that." But most ladies will require some sort of clitoral or potentially vaginal incitement to oblige that if they need to experience the heavenly pleasure too.

Rest climax

We've had arousing dreams previously. Be that as it may, this is an entirely another thing. "A few ladies can have a climax during a suggestive dream while resting," says Dr. Ross. One report demonstrates that 37% of ladies have had one of these rest climaxes when they're 45, yet it's hard to tell how basic they truly are.

Rest climaxes for the most part start with an attractive dream, which causes expanded bloodstream to the private parts just as significant unwinding, which some way or another enables the body to arrive at climax while a lady isn't conscious.

Various climaxes

You can't have an overdose of something that is otherwise good, isn't that so? That is the intrigue of various climaxes, something ladies can enjoy because not at all like men, females don't encounter a hard-headed period in the wake of peaking that requires some personal time before preparing for cycle two.

Ladies arrive at a certain uplifted condition of joy with their first climax and after that can keep awake there on this level. With increasingly more incitement, they can have numerous climaxes. Numerous ladies do encounter this, she says, yet only one out of every odd lady will need to.

However, if you do, here's a technique: continue getting your pelvic muscles without anyone else (by pressing and discharging how you would if you were holding in your pee stream), recommends Dr. Corridor. This keeps the bloodstream high, which builds affectability and makes climax number 2 simpler to reach. If you don't go right down to the pre-excitement state, you can stir your way up to another climax all the more rapidly.

Male orgasm

Ways to give him the best orgasm
Even though it appears to be straightforward enough, the male climax is an unpredictable procedure. Men accomplish climax through a progression of steps including various organs, hormones, veins, and nerves cooperating. The regular outcome is a discharge of liquid that may contain sperm through solid muscle contractions. Let us take a gander at the manners in which that will cause him to have an immense amazing climax.

One caution before we start: Be set up for shocks, and for appearing inconsistencies. Things being what they are, male climaxes are both as resolute as they now and then appear, and simultaneously significantly progressively confounded. As touchy as men are to aptitude and procedure, they're similarly controlled by the state of mind, time and the condition, and timing. It will be fun for partners if you combine the following strategies to enhance an amazing orgasm for him.

Express your immense love for him

The greatest mystery about men's climaxes is that they uncover their weakness. That is the reason they're so touchy to the earth; slight changes in the breeze can transform a 10-firearm salute into a popgun. A few men state that some of the time think that it's hard to cum at all if he's also stressed over his activity.

The shock while talking with men to write this was that just one of them said he appreciated being brought to climax through oral sex. That is a road I expected would be number one on most men's hit procession. Also, it is nevertheless just as foreplay.

Men are truly searching for very similar things from sex that ladies are: love, acknowledgment, and closeness. The snapshot of climax is the point at which those requirements are most uncovered, and men even wedded men — can get apprehensive being sincerely stripped. At the point when asked what procedures delivered his most serious climaxes, one man affectionately reviewed sweethearts who snatched him by his butt and pulled him more tightly toward them, as though they don't need anything to such an extent as to assimilate him.

Jason, a 40-year-old official, discussed how his significant other some of the time affectionately does the stroking of his face as he comes. "It's about her demonstrating that she truly needs me," he says. Specialists can speak for quite a long time about how to accomplish genuine closeness, however, a decent spot to begin would be sleeping today. Tell your man the amount you adore him, and would not joke about this. At that point hang on with a death grip.

Give him a treat by taking charge during the night

A decent climax for a man is what could be compared to a cool lager toward the part of the bargain: a delightful reward for occupation all around done. The activity for this situation is satisfying you. A noteworthy piece of the fulfillment men get from sex is the self-image support that outcomes from causing our accomplices to go bonkers in bed.

The fact of the matter is that a lot of men won't enable themselves to enjoy their very own climax until they've achieved that objective. The aim is to perform first and get to the climax as the second goal. There are times when men simply need to come, however essentially their objective is for the partner to locate each sexual experience thoroughly satisfying.

Sex advisers will disclose to you that even though this methodology is splendid better that men be excessively worried about their accomplices' climaxes than not in any way concerned — it can regardless comprise a type of intentional tactile hardship. By getting control over their enthusiasm, numerous men deny themselves of the sexual relinquish that creates the most grounded climaxes. According to sex, therapist Sex turns into a fight to ensure she has a climax, instead of a common sharing of happiness.

Here is what you should do about it. Let your man relax by taking control of the night. Urge him to concentrate on living it up without stressing over dealing with you. There are two essential approaches to this. One is to let him know, as your lovemaking warms up, that you need this one to be supportive of him, that today he ought to do whatever makes him feel better. The other is to urge him to lie back latently and let himself be pleasured by you. Sex advisers state this is a superior strategy since it empowers him to focus totally on what he's an inclination, as opposed to on what he's doing. The equivalent ought to go for you when he gives back where its due one more night: Ideally, both of you will routinely alternate showing the other magnificent exercises in the craft of orgasmic appreciation. A marriage therapist says numerous men think that it's hard to relinquish control during sex. Try not to be astounded, at that point, on the off chance that it takes some time before your significant other is open to turning the reins totally over to you. Be understanding, yet be firm. He'll figure out how to adore it.

Tease him occasionally

Ask any man following seven days out and about forbearance is the world's most dominant sexual enhancer. Notwithstanding when he's not away, you can add to that repressed, kicking the bucket to-have intercourse perspective by conveying some sexual prodding strategies during the day. A sex specialist recommends incidentally blazing a little bosom at him in the first part of the day or giving him a prurient telephone call at the workplace. Further, it is uncovered ladies can plant a sexual seed that will bloom that night into a more grounded climax.

Keep stroking him

A similar drive that makes a man become a creature when he returns home from an excursion is grinding away inside every individual episode of lovemaking. During foreplay, muscle strain fabricates and the genital zone ends up engorged with blood, bringing about a consistently developing weight for discharge. The more weight, the more joy in the discharge, because the withdrawals tend either to be more grounded or last more.

In our true inner being, we men realize that the more drawn out the foreplay, the more grounded the climax, for ourselves just as for our accomplices. And yet, we have this amazingly ground-breaking drive to just come, come, come! We can't resist: It's been designed into our sexual hardware more than a large number of years.

The stunt for you is to enable your significant other to put aside this transformative goal with the goal that sex endures long enough for a momentous peak to construct. There is a recommendation that establishing the pace for more, progressively languorous sex by beginning things off with a moderate, exotic back rub. Other postponing strategies can be brought into play as the merriments progress. Halting for an infrequent chilling period works delightfully, yet takes discipline.

The lady on-top position is valuable since it enables the man to control his desire to begin pushing. A delaying strategy that may take practice is known as the "press system." Just before his climax seems inescapable, put your thumb on one side of the base of the penis and the tips of your list and center fingers on the opposite side, at that point crush. You would then be able to begin your shared climb to the peak once more.

Surprise him

A result of the fast in and out of the idea is the sneak assault: A component of sexual astonishment can deliver an incredible peak. Now and then you have to slice through all the confusion and mess of current life. Anything from employment weight to cash misfortunes to kid issues to room weariness can separate you and your man's most profound interests. Immediacy can help carry him to his detects. A decent time to attempt this is on the morning of the weekend. That is typically when men are most loose the level for and their testosterone is at the climax.

It's not so much politically right to concede this, however in all actuality when the climax is up and coming, there's just a single male erogenous zone, and you know where it is. "That doesn't mean men don't care to be kissed or touched, yet with regards to climax, you can begin and end with the penis.

It bodes well, subsequently, when men are looking for the best orgasm, their places of the decision will, in general, be those that give the most immediate penile incitement, and the best open doors for the penile push. "For unadulterated physicality, the back passage is the best approach. There's more erosion, more profundity. I likewise adore it when my significant other is on top, holding herself up, particularly when she does that retrogressive."

Carl likewise refers to another most loved type of penile incitement: the vaginal crush of a lady who's been doing her Kegel works out. Kegels fortify the PC muscle, the one you grasp when you need to close off your progression of pee. Out of the blue, it feels like a hand holding you and that feels astonishing.

Drive him nuts with a creative quickie

Excitement is a strange and amazing thing, and some of the time the furious forsake of a fast and obscene coupling can deliver a peak that is just as dangerous as a long-distance race session in the sack. I speculate this has something to do with that hundreds of years old sexual hardware we referenced: Sex without function can take advantage of profound repositories of creature nature. One man recalls when he had perhaps the most grounded climax when his partner overwhelmed him as he guiltlessly returned home from work one night — bits of apparel were dissipated between the front entryway and the room. I'm certain the way that she was the creative stoked the flame.

Contact the illegal zones

As focused as we men are on our penises, there are other key spots that, when invigorated, can send us lurching over the edge. A few men state that having their gonads out of this world elevates the feeling. Ladies are more stressed over contacting the gonads than they ought to be. It's just when you slam into the gonads that it harms. Having the scrotum scoured feels incredible. Other touchy spots appear to depend more on close to home taste. Men cherish it when their significant other rubs his titties; Another man reviews a sweetheart who voraciously sucked his fingers.

If he's alright with butt-centric play, a prostate back rub can bring about an extra serious, delayed climax. To discover his, gradually embed a well-lubed finger around one inch into his butt, at that point move your digit in a "come here" movement.
Find other sweet spots
There are parts all over a person's body that may invigorate him and make him insane – and they might be more subtle than the previously mentioned spots. Have you given any

thought to his middle, sanctuaries, or chest? All things considered, you should.

P spot

There is the delicate space between his balls and butt. Simply applying strain to invigorate the perineum can uplift a male climax. Regardless of the situating, arrive at an arm around or through to tenderly put a fingertip or even knuckle on the territory, taking consideration to perceive how he responds to check whether that weight is correct.

Talk dirty

Have you considered all the hot things you can say to a man? Spoiler alert: The dirtier, the better. Try not to think little of the power your words can have during foreplay, paving the way to something much progressively hazardous for him.

Be focused on the moment

The male climax comprises of two phases. In stage 1, the sperm is drawn up from the balls and pooled with ejaculatory liquids in a kind of organizing territory just beneath the prostate organ. Bosses and Johnson called this the purpose of "ejaculatory certainty," implying that the man's mom, his minister, and his previous sweetheart could stroll in the room, and his climax would proceed as though nothing had occurred. Stage 2, comes in seconds later after the fact, is discharged.

On the off chance that conceivable, abstain from intruding on your man's fixation as the stages unfurl. Utilizing strategies that both of you know and like is fine, yet surprising, emotional moves at the purpose of climax are bound to divert than a highlight. Moving a great deal falls into that class. Essentially remain back, so to speak, and let his climax occur. It's not an opportunity to get extravagant or imaginative. Once more, a situation: How would you find better approaches to push your man over the top without interfering with his orgasmic fixation? Understand that you need to pick a few evenings to analysis and others to go for the pinnacle involvement.

Be playful with his body

Running your fingers through your man's chest hair probably won't appear as though it does a ton, yet that is the place you'd not be right the region is delicate to such an extent that this straightforward demonstration can drive him wild. Spot your hand level on their lower chest or gut and, keeping your palm on their skin, run it up to their chest until you have a bunch of hair. Pull, beginning tenderly pulling along these lines animates the nerve endings without giving that parsimonious hair-pulling feel. You can do this on their head, as well, beginning at the back of their neck.

Be mindful

It's a trendy expression for stress help and reflection, yet care is tied in with valuing the present minute and the majority of its sensations. That can be intense during the harsh and-tumble activity of sex. "Have a go at ensuring that the other individual remains in their body during sex, and truly encounters the joy," rather than daydreaming or notwithstanding losing themselves in it, says Blaylock-Johnson. "You're not progressing in the direction of climax, yet simply being available."

You can try different things with your very own care, or get him to your attractive Zen headspace by keeping in touch, easing back your breathing, and keeping your developments drowsy.

The magical Socks

It sounds positively unsexy, yet one investigation discovered it can make your intimacy significantly more smoking. Scientists at the University of Groningen discovered 80% of couples had the option to have a climax while wearing socks contrasted with only half without socks. So perhaps whenever you get stripped, leave on simply that one thing of apparel.

Take all control

An increasingly outrageous adaptation of expanding the foreplay is designated "edging," where you get him straight up to the truth, edge, and afterward back off. You stop before you experience peak, and stew, at that point rehash that a couple of times. It develops the vitality with the goal that you have a progressively, well, touchy and exceptional climax. Obviously, let him know whether that is your arrangement, else he may very well believe you're being mean.

Chapter 4

Sexual health

Concocting a meaning of sexual well-being is a troublesome undertaking, as each culture, sub-culture, and individual has various principles of sexual well-being. Sexual well-being is the capacity to grasp and make the most of our sexuality for the duration of our lives. It is a significant piece of our physical and enthusiastic well-being. Being explicitly sound methods:

Getting to know that sexuality is a characteristic piece of life and includes more than sexual conduct

Perceiving and regarding the sexual rights we as a whole connect with.

Approaching sexual well-being data, training, and care

Attempting to anticipate unintended pregnancies and STDs and look for consideration and treatment when required.

Having the option to encounter sexual joy, fulfillment, and closeness when wanted

Importance of sexual health

The expression "sexual well-being" envelops a scope of general well-being and clinical issues identified with the counteractive action of explicitly transmitted contaminations. I utilize the expression a ton in my very own work and its broadening cash is a welcome new worldview in our field. Truth be told, the idea of sexual well-being appears to be of central significance to all parts of the aversion of explicitly transmitted contaminations.

To be completely forthright, however, the majority of the discussions about sexual well-being doesn't appear to have affected the everyday points of interest in our work. Sex still is fundamentally observed as a lot of hazard factors that we counsel against. I am persuaded that this point of view on sex and sexuality as "chance" legitimates the disgrace related with explicitly transmitted diseases and adds to our general public's toxic narrow mindedness of sexual assorted variety. A sexual well-being viewpoint fuses the idea of individual and epidemiologic dangers of sex however perceives the inescapable significance of sex in our lives.

In any case, I've started to think about whether I comprehend what sexual well-being implies in any case. It's a major idea, and possibly it's regular that definitions appear to be hopeful, exhausted, and pompous. Consider the notable working meaning of the World Health Organization:

"Sexual well being is a condition of physical, enthusiastic, mental and social prosperity in connection to sexuality; it isn't simply the nonappearance of sickness, brokenness or ailment. Sexual well-being requires a positive and aware way to deal with sexuality and sexual connections, just as the plausibility of having pleasurable and safe sexual encounters, free of pressure, separation, and savagery. For sexual well-being to be accomplished and kept up, the sexual privileges of all people must be regarded, secured and satisfied."

There is a ton to concur inside this definition, particularly in its acknowledgment of the complex physical, passionate, mental and social properties of sexual well-being, and the tying down of sexual well-being in widespread sexual rights. Be that as it may, I see this definition as interestingly scolding and parental. All the more critically, be that as it may, the definition is explicitly dubious. Regardless of how often I've perused, utilized, and referred to this definition, I can't get from it even a simple vision of how sexual well-being works in individuals' day by day lives. I feel the equivalent about the more as of late created meaning of the Places for Disease Control and Prevention, especially because sexual rights and of sexual joy are missing from that sexual well-being definition.

Thus, perhaps I have to get more clear with myself about what sexual well-being is. Also, sexual well-being ought to be something other than the negatives: not pressured; not segregated; not savage. The predominance of these negatives in numerous individuals' lives discloses to us how far we are from accomplishing a fair and impartial society. In any case, I imagine that sexual well-being, at last, requires substantially more dynamic association from us all, and it appears to be very inadequate to trust that sexual well-being will emerge alone if intimidation, segregation, and viciousness are at long last prevailed.

Sexual well-being is a major piece of life. It can influence and is influenced by different parts of well-being. This incorporates physical, mental, enthusiastic, and social well-being. Being in great sexual well-being implies you are all around educated, cautious, and aware of yourself as well as other people. It likewise means living it up explicitly in a manner you are OK with.

Way to prosperity

Training

A great many people find out about sexuality and sex from the get-go. You may have dialogues with guardians, kin, educators, or guides. Or on the other hand, you may find it all alone. You find out about sexual orientation and genitalia. You find out about what sex is and the dangers it conveys. Dangers incorporate pregnancy, explicitly transmitted diseases (STIs), and sexual maltreatment. It is critical to learn as much as you can about sex. The more educated you are, the more set you up are to use sound judgment.

Well-being

There are numerous approaches to secure your sexual well-being and care for yourself. Forbearance is the best way to 100% forestall pregnancy and STIs. This implies not having vaginal, butt-centric, or oral sex.

On the off chance that you choose to be explicitly dynamic, you might need to think about a type of conception prevention. Various sorts incorporate a condom, pill, fix, shot, embed, stomach, or intrauterine gadget (IUD). These can help anticipate undesirable pregnancy. Condoms are the main strategy to help avert STIs.

Converse with your primary care physician before you start engaging in sexual relations. They will converse with you progressively about security, dangers, and anticipation. They can respond to any inquiries you have about sexual well-being. They additionally can recommend a type of conception prevention.

A few people have sexual issues or limitations. Certain meds and conditions can restrict want or capacity. Converse with your primary care physician before you assume control on drugs, or if you have reactions, for example, torment, from sex.

Correspondence

Another piece of sexual well-being is correspondence. Discussion about sex to a specialist, parent, or grown-up you trust. It is ideal to be straightforward with inquiries and worries.

You additionally should be immediate and clear with the accomplice you are explicitly keen on. Discussion about your desires and set limits. Try not to let the person in question or different companions, weight you into anything. You should just do things that you concur, or assent, too. Try not to accomplish something that you would prefer not to do or that makes you awkward. If you wind up in a circumstance like this, tell the individual "no." Then leave the circumstance and educate somebody you trust regarding it. They can secure you and get you help, if necessary.

On the off chance that you have been determined to have an STI, you should tell your sexual partner(s). They might be influenced also. The more accomplices you have, the higher your danger of getting an STI. Treatment can help fix or soothe the side effects of some STIs.

Interesting points

It is typical for your sexual well-being to develop as you age. To remain sound, it is ideal to routinely consider your contemplations, sentiments, and feelings. Doing this ahead of time will set you up for sexual experiences.

Sexual wellbeing isn't something you ought to oversee individually. It is something you should discuss with individuals you trust or love. You can discuss what is viewed as sheltered and what the dangers are of sure activities. You ought to comprehend what assent is and that it's alright to state "no."

On the off chance that you think of pregnancy, having an STI infection, or have been manhandled, look for assistance immediately. For pregnancy and STIs, a specialist can do a test to affirm. They can give you more data and examine your choices. For maltreatment, a specialist can perform tests and give treatment. A cop or legal advisor can give lawful help. You likewise might need to see an instructor, who can offer passionate help.

Inquiries to pose to your primary care physician

In what manner will I know whether I'm prepared to have intercourse?

What are the dangers of having intercourse?

If I choose to engage in sexual relations, should I be on contraception?

How might I practice sex that is safe?

Are there any antibodies I ought to get before I have intercourse?

I had intercourse, however now I wish I hadn't. What would I be able to do?

How would I know whether I am in poor sexual well-being?

What would it be advisable for me to do in case I'm worried about my sexual well-being?

When there is no functioning in the bedroom

In various gatherings with partners, there has been constant communication on foreplay.

Normally, men prepare for sex in a flash, particularly in their initial a long time in a relationship. Ladies, then again, need to experience readiness.

Solid sexuality necessitates that the lady is decidedly ready and that she is free of torment during sex. This can't occur except if there is sufficient oil. Oil happens when there is an ideal foreplay.

One of the normal issues making ladies and men visit a sexologist today is wounds after sex. The wounds are not confined to the lady; men also get them because of dry sex. "Is there a likelihood that I could be irregular?" Jane asked, "Are there ladies who simply get telephone calls from their life partners and grease up normally in an arrangement without being contacted?"

All things considered, in ordinary conditions, sex accomplices need to sentiment before they are prepared for penetrative sex. It is irregular that a lady would get grease through a telephone call.

Reflecting, I noticed that Jane's pickle was a sign of a more serious issue that youthful couples experience today. Individuals engage in sexual relations with no abilities since society has not created frameworks for causing them to learn. Gone are the days when youngsters and ladies would sit with their aunts, uncles, and grandparents to find out about sex. Today individuals find out about sex from TV and sentimental books and magazines. A large portion of what they gain from these channels is ridiculous since it is generally dramatization and different types of acting. The outcome is that individuals have strange minds about sex as they get seeing someone.

"All around put specialist. Along these lines, what must we do to cure this circumstance?" Jane asked when I met her with her significant other at the center.

Without people group frameworks that can show us sex, it is profoundly suggested that couples go for sex advising by a certified sexologist or sexual medicine specialist. Again you must be cautious because there are many phony specialists in the market. Qualified sexual well-being experts confer aptitudes that are pivotal for solid and palatable sex.

For a quick arrangement, I endorsed a grease for Jane as the couple experienced sex instructing. Ointments are fake gels used to enhance normal grease. There are circumstances like Jane's the place for some explanation characteristic oil neglects to occur. The lady applies an ointment before sex to stay away from results of dry sex. The underlying driver of dry sex must, in any case, be dealt with so the lady can grease up normally.

It is imperative to take note of that an extraordinary oil or cream can be utilized for grease. Utilizing glycerin, for instance, can prompt rehashed candida diseases. Prescribed ointments are characterized into either water-based or silicone oils or a blend of the two. Water-based greases evaporate inside 15 minutes while silicon ointments take hours to evaporate. A blend of the two gives a couple of sufficient time to have their pleasure. When purchasing a grease, discover what it is made of.

"I am of the lube specialist and the injuries are gone," said Jane half a month after our first experience. She and her significant other had been experiencing sex instructing and had aced the specialty of foreplay. Jane had the option to grease up normally and didn't require the "lube" any longer.

PHYSICAL INTIMACY

Physical closeness is described by kinship, non-romantic love, sentimental love, or sexual movement. While there are a few unique sorts of closeness, physical closeness is just one of those. It is regularly about sex, yet considerably more. Association and correspondence with others around us manufacture physical closeness and regularly, fascination in somebody of the contrary sex is the key marker of physical closeness.

The incorporation of physical closeness in human sexuality is another factor that requires thought. It is accounted for that a great many people want physical closeness or something to that effect in any event at times, being that it is a characteristic piece of human sexuality. Since this is regularly exotic contacting of any kind, it requires a passage into another's close to home space, while it might be an enthusiastic or sexual act anyplace from an embrace to a kiss or sex. Passionate or sexy contacting of this sort helps in the arrival of oxytocin, dopamine, and serotonin, which diminishes pressure. Additionally, without physical closeness, there are expanded sentiments of depression or pity.

It is intriguing to realize that many explanations to closeness and enthusiasm don't separate between the two, or genuinely separate sexual closeness from the theme. There is a general theme of a personal relationship. There is an understanding that every one of these things can be consolidated in the closeness between two individuals further their relationship develops. Physical associations like sex and enthusiastic associations likewise incorporate love and relational relations.

Cozy connections exist between two individuals with physical or enthusiastic closeness. While the term personal relationship, as a rule, suggests the incorporation of sexual action, the term is additionally used to demonstrate an association with something other than sexual movement. Personal connections keep up a key job in the general human experience since they include passionate associations with others. This might be a sentiment, physical or sexual fascination, sexual movement, or enthusiastic help, while additionally helping individuals create solid relational associations.

All in all, the inquiry exists, "Are sex and closeness various things?" We may likewise ask, "Would you be able to have each separately? Or on the other hand, does one lead to another?" There are many clashing assessments on the jobs of sex and closeness inside and outside of connections. Since no two individuals have similar thoughts on sex, there is no limited response to any of these issues. In a customary structure, sex incorporates long haul duty or marriage, trailed by enthusiastic closeness and multiplication. Nonetheless, in an inexorably wanton society, the association between sex and closeness can be a shaky one.

What does sexual passion entail

Presently, this might be as straightforward as solace with individual fondness or with open showcases of warmth as a result of the degree of closeness that has created between two individuals. There is likewise the topic of whether there is sex or sexual enthusiasm without feeling or love, and whether it very well may be kept up.

Strikingly enough, when searching for the meaning of sexual enthusiasm, a large number of indistinguishable references from physical closeness showed up in various word reference areas. One extra notice is that of "fondness," something that is of expansion to the physical contacting and closeness that accompanies the feelings being communicated. While "love" and "love" are not the equivalent, this demonstrates there might be something more enthusiastic in the energetic side of this word blend.

Individuals who are close and commonplace are increasingly open to entering each other's close to home space and taking on physical contact. Contingent upon the relationship, open presentations of friendship may fluctuate dependent on the social standard in which they get themselves. These presentations can extend from straightforward motions like a kiss or embrace to a grasp or clasping hands. While this might be a straightforward welcome, there might be long haul contact or tender grasp kept up in the open space when these two individuals are very alright with one another.

At that point, there are techniques for contact that are kept up in private in a progressively personal relationship. As two individuals become more like each other they are calm and can show types of affections when together including:

Snuggling

Stroking

Tickling

Backrub

Contacting or entwining of legs

These occasions don't require sexual action to have energy or closeness, yet this would almost certainly show that it's anything but an explicitly energetic relationship. On the off chance that two individuals are hoping to keep up fellowship, it is more probable they will adhere to an embrace or kiss on the cheek to show care or warmth that isn't explicitly enthusiastic.

Consequently, physical sexual closeness can differ in the definition. A few people are more explicitly enthusiastic than others and can bring that degree of closeness into a sentimental relationship considerably more effectively. There is additionally the way that every individual sees sex, in any event, a somewhat extraordinary way, and usually, people unexpectedly address sexual closeness and enthusiasm.

Difference between sex and intimacy

Sex with no affection or closeness is an inquiry that is at the center of any solid relationship. Since there is the estimation of sex between two individuals who have a personal or adoring relationship, there is likewise the significance of characterizing every single distinctive bit of the relationship. General closeness includes knowing somebody profoundly and the capacity to feel open, free and fair with them. This is something that is regularly just felt or experienced with one individual, as this nearby closeness is too hard to even think about having with numerous individuals.

In this way, sex in a cherishing or private relationship will, in general, be the physical exemplification of those emotions. The perfect hypothesis is that this physical closeness is to be a cherishing association between the two individuals in a relationship. Both of them inside a relationship is in this manner interconnected: physical closeness manufactures sexual enthusiasm, and sexual energy constructs sexual closeness.

There is the capacity to isolate sexual energy from physical closeness also. This is if sex is only a physical demonstration, particularly when it happens outside of a relationship. Inside a relationship, sex is the most private act, yet there are various events when this demonstration can happen. It tends to be a physical demonstration that happens without assent (assault), a demonstration that is paid for (prostitution), or a straightforward physical trade (one-night stand).

State that we consider the one-night stands that anybody takes on following a night of drinking or celebrating with companions. Any man or lady can appreciate a night of sex without adoration or closeness, more often than not when there is a physical fascination or the fundamental want for happiness regarding sex. It is frequently a mental inquiry of the distinction between these two, and the general close and helpless demonstration of offering yourself to another in sex, which would interface both sex and closeness once more.

When the assurance of sexual energy or physical closeness is made, there then comes the topic of sex or having intercourse. With this having been a solid discussion for extensive periods, there is the possibility to comprehend this is an autonomous choice to be made. Or if nothing else this would be the chosen term between the two accomplices who have set up their close, sexual relationship.

Since regardless of the term utilized, sex is constantly a physical demonstration and should be possible without closeness. Notwithstanding, there is the potential for the love or closeness engaged with this demonstration to be a degree or level of association-related between the two accomplices included, making it something that turns out to be progressively cozy or increasingly a type of lovemaking as their relationship develops after some time.

It is likewise essential to recollect that cherishing and private couples on occasion can't have intercourse or decide not to do as such. There can be ailments that forestall sex, making the physical closeness in their relationship something of a milder level. This doesn't dispose of the enthusiasm or fascination they feel for each other. It additionally doesn't evacuate different types of physical closeness and contacting, or quality time spent together to express their affection and feelings for each other.

ANAL SEX

The passionate suggestion you feel before boarding a crazy ride is about equivalent to you feel directly before setting out on butt-centric sex: fervor, trailed by mellow wavering and anxiety. Be that as it may! The thing about every roller coaster ride I've been on (up until now) is that I've cherished them all. Regardless of what several butterflies are tap-moving on the base of my stomach as the ride sways up a lofty slope, the rush I feel toward the part of the bargain is constantly justified, despite all the trouble.

It is not necessarily the case that everybody who preferences exciting rides will likewise like butt-centric sex. The takeaway from this allegory is that it's especially fine to be anxious about it in advance—regardless of whether you're certain (and you ought to be), this is something you need to do.

Butt-centric sex requires a touch of additional readiness, however other than that, it's simply one more sex act.

Regardless of whether despite everything you're bantering to get in line for this specific thrill ride, or areas of now staggering up the precarious slope, here's all that you have to think about butt-centric sex.

All that you should know on anal sex

1. Try not to attempt it on the off chance that you would prefer not to. There's a major distinction between "I don't fantasize about getting a penis douche yet I need to take my accomplice's breath away" and "I would prefer to bite the dust than do this yet I surmise I can endure it since he's been influencing me." If you're in a commonly minding, solid relationship (with a person who goes down on you for thirty minutes, least), perhaps you'll need to do it for your accomplice or you won't. Whichever way is okay, and on the off chance that he continues forcing you when you have clarified that it isn't on the table, instruct him to suck it.

2. Evaluate butt-centric play first. Before leaving on the full mount of penetrative, butt-centric sex, you can—and should! try lighter butt-centric play out. This is available to understanding and could mean anything from toys to fingers or mouths. It'll give you a lower-weight thought of what the ~sensations~ of butt-centric incitement feel like, and is a method for working up to the huge show. Or on the other hand

not! If you choose some light butt-centric play is all, you're keen on, stay outdoors there until the end of time. No guidelines here, but to utilize lube, have assent and make use of lube.

3. On the off chance that it harms, stop! A few, well, we should call them new sensations are not out of the ordinary—a lot of ladies state it feels like they have to crap, or like a basic, weight feeling. In any case, similar to some other sex act, if things begin to hurt such that is never again fun, you should stop. Wounds from butt-centric sex are conceivable, however overly uncommon. Agony most ordinarily originates from butt-centric crevices, or little tears in the tissue around the rear-end, which is extremely meager and fragile. A decent method to cure that is utilizing heaps of lube and hurting with littler articles, instead of enormous ones.

4. You may drain a bit. As usual, in case you're draining abundantly or perseveringly (like, for longer than 60 minutes), you should call a specialist. In any case, a little blood during butt-centric play or sex isn't irregular. Study reveals that the most widely recognized explanation behind seeping after butt-centric sex is butt-centric tears little tears or crevices in the sensitive butt-centric trench tissue. Before you oddity out at the idea of "butt-centric tears," realize that a large portion of these is so little you won't feel them, and a great deal of them

don't create any blood whatsoever. However, similar to snowflakes, no two butt-centric tears are the equivalent, so yours may drain a piece. These little folks ought to recuperate inside a couple of days yet may cause a touch of mellow uneasiness when you're crapping.

Another extremely basic reason is hemorrhoid (that is correct, we're talkin' hemorrhoids, people) you didn't think about. This is more disturbing because hemorrhoid holds a lot of blood inside. You'll likely feel some degree of inconvenience or agony on the off chance that you have hemorrhoid, and if it blasts, you'll unquestionably observe some draining that ought to thoroughly die down inside a couple of days.

5. You're going to be vocal during this procedure. Regardless of whether you're typically exceptionally calm during sex, this is a period you'll wanna shout out—particularly your first time giving it a shot with another accomplice. Let them know whether they're going excessively quick, on the off chance that you have an inclination that you're going to crap all over, or in case you're encountering torment/uneasiness. Additionally, let them know whether it feels better! In case you're feeling anxious, odds are your accomplice is, as well. Positive input— we adore it!

6. Toss other incitement in with the general mish-mash. Tune in, they don't make those wild-looking, three-pronged sex toys to no end. When you're ready of things, include some clit incitement, some vaginal incitement, or hell, each of the three. A few ladies state this combo feels overstimulating in the most ideal manner. Regardless, most ladies need a mix of incitement to climax—whether that is clit/vaginal, or butt-centric/clit+vaginal is abstract. However, would it say it isn't enjoyable to adapt to new things about your climaxes?

7. Regardless of whether you're monogamous, a condom is presumably a smart thought. It keeps microscopic organisms from the insides spreading anyplace. Having wipes on the end table and to not utilize a similar condom going from vaginal to butt-centric and back again.

8. The correct lube is twice as significant as it is when having vaginal sex, which is super-significant. You may have heard that a lot of lube removes the grinding that makes it feel useful for the fella. That is horse crap. There is nothing of the sort as a lot of lube since it makes it feel marginally less like you are utilizing your butthole as a tote for an electric lamp.

9. Between slight water-based, lubes and thicker ones (KY), go with the thicker ones, since they don't dry out as fast. In sex there is an insane useful Ultimate Guide to Anal Sex for

Women, she refers to that Crisco has been a most loved of the LGBT people group for quite a while, however, it's terrible to use with condoms since it can in the long run jab modest gaps in the latex.

there are those with oil which are additionally really irritating to get off a short time later. We utilized Vaseline, yet my sweetheart later understood that it stifles sensation on the skin, which was useful for my butt head however awful for his climax. So perhaps don't do that, or start with a touch of that however then switch, since it'll take truly long for your accomplice to come on the off chance that they are able.

10. Getting the tip in damages the most because the leader of the penis is the amplest part. When you're past that and up to the pole, it'll feel somewhat better. Keep in mind what amount of standard sex hurt from the outset, for a few of us?

11. Loosen up the muscles of your personal computer however much as could be expected. Unwinding and contracting the pubococcygeus (PC) muscles resembles the butt-centric form of doing Kegels. You can stress over that later on — at this moment simply let your butthole muscles go, similar to you're going to crap (you won't, most likely).

12. You're going to crack the fuck out that you're crapping yet you're most certainly not. Truly, it turns out to be difficult to discern whether you are or aren't; moreover, this Tucker Max story was not useful for my butt sex-fear. You're most likely not going to crap. If there's a smidgen of crap, as my accomplice stated, it is anything but a major ordeal, because "[he] requested this." (There wasn't.)

13. The positions you can try are relaxing on your stomach, get in doggy-style, or do teacher—and that is the request for what will hurt the least to the most. In any event, as far as I can tell. You can tear your butt if you utilize a specific position that takes into account more entrance before you're prepared, and Taormino brings up that the evangelist position takes into consideration the least clitoral incitement and proposes collector on-top for learners. "Insertive accomplices who are unpracticed, anxious about how to enter their accomplices anally, or dreadful of harming their accomplices may discover this position most unwinding because the collector can do a significant part of the basic leadership and work."

Try not to stress over disillusioning him by needing to go moderate and delicately. You're not being a buzzkill who's squashing his pornography impacted dreams of beating the poo out of a young lady's butt. You are being a magnificent and caring partner if anal sex isn't on your rundown of must-have intercourse.

Chapter 5

Sexual fantasy

Everybody has sexual dreams once in a while. What's more, as it's been said, regardless of what you envision, another person has thought about it in any event once. Be that as it may, progressing from a position of the creative mind to finishing on your wants can be precarious. That is the place sex specialists come in, with certain stunts for seeking after sexual dreams that may dispel any confusion air as you make sense of what you need in bed.

As a matter of first importance, there's nothing amiss with your dream being something that you either can't or don't have any desire to, carry on. "Dream is free space. It doesn't generally bode well and it doesn't need to," sexologist and relationship master Dr. Nikki Goldstein tells Bustle. If you have sexual dreams that incorporate anything especially risky or illicit, it's feasible best to talk about it with an expert. Be that as it may, on the off chance that your dream is just innovative or somewhat forbidden, at that point there's an opportunity it may be something worth seeking after with somebody happy to investigate it also.

The society has developed negativities on sex, there can be somewhat of a hazy area around whether it's you who doesn't need this plan to work out as intended, or whether you're simply apprehensive. So it's essential to separate it a piece. When you do, you can realize in the case of something is a dream or an all-out want. "Want is something you long to do. A dream is only an idea," Goldstein says. Also, if it's extremely something beyond an idea, you have the right to know.

Here are eight different ways to separate between a dream and something you truly need in bed, as indicated by specialists.

Decide to actualize the fantasy
The most significant advance is just bringing your dream into the setting. "Consider doing it in consistently life. "Does regardless it appear to be engaging and energizing?"

Regardless of whether it be unadulterated coordination or the way that your dream includes non-monogamy when you're in a submitted relationship, in some cases a dream simply doesn't make it past this progression. "A dream may have components of heavenly or anecdotal characters. It may include time travel or superhuman quality. It may very well be something that serenely lives in an individual's mind and they want to feel on or in their body. A longing talks more to envisioning this thing truly occurring, and it's sensible, in any event to a degree, and the sorcerer is OK with any results." If you can without much of a stretch say that your dream sounds great in a genuine setting, at that point you're likely a bit nearer to getting it going.

Check whether there are negative impacts

This progression fundamentally includes posing yourself one inquiry: do you have more to lose, or to pick up, on the off chance that you finish on this? Consider the ramifications of experienced that dream. "Does it include other individuals? How might an accomplice respond? Would it risk the relationship?" Each piece of this greater answer will give you added signs to whether this dream has a place in your sexual coexistence.

Then again, on the off chance that you have a feeling that you have something to lose by not finishing on this present, that is a major sign as well. "If you have a dream that is a consistent wellspring of suggestive vitality and warmth and it would squash you not to appreciate it, hold off and attempt to make sense of how, at any rate, to enhance the examination. Regardless of whether it appears to be a piece nerve-wracking, if you can't deal with keeping this in your mind any more (and it's protected, consensual, and legitimate), it's most likely simply time to put it all on the line.

Actualize the date for the trial

Simply set a date for the dream situation, and afterward perceive how you feel as the date draws near. "On the off chance that you are energized, energetic, and grinning, it's likely something you need to do in bed. On the off chance that there is anxiety, if you delay, on the off chance that you experience fear or frenzy, it's reasonable a dream that should remain as such. Along these lines, you'll have the option to abstain from getting excessively near something that you would not like to do, and become familiar with yourself for what's to come.

Discussion with someone about it

It might be nerve-wracking, yet it is OK to discuss sex with others. Furthermore, an ever-increasing number of individuals are getting settled with the subject, as well, so you likely won't be the main individual you know to get open about the subject.

Simply raising the subject around a companion may open up certain considerations or emotions you were beforehand unfit to reveal. Also, if your discussion with companions doesn't support enough, you can generally look for different types of assistance, as well. On the off chance that an individual is truly confounded, at that point converse with an instructor about it.

Numerous individuals come to me to work out what is a dream that should remain similarly as a dream and what might be conceivable to investigate. No issue who you wind up opening up to, it'll likely be a decent advance towards understanding your sexuality on a more profound level.

Check if your accomplice is intrigued

If your dream is anything but a performance demonstration, at that point, you're going to need to think about the other individual (or individuals) included. For a great many people this exhibits the best issue.

Fortunately, in case you're single or non-monogamous, access to the Internet and distinctive applications means you're almost certain than any time in recent memory to discover somebody into indistinguishable things from you. What's more, on the off chance that you have one accomplice, now and again simply discussing the thought can be provocative in itself.

It's essential to likewise take note of that a dream can be a pointer that you may require an adjustment in your sexual coexistence. Some of the time this step implies seeking after the dream and leaving your previous existence to do as such. If somebody always fantasizes about individuals of an unexpected sexual orientation in comparison to them, for the most part, join forces with that may mean they're attempting to turn out as gay or promiscuous, for example. Listening to your dreams could mean a noteworthy life advance.

Try the easy version

Regardless of whether all signs point to "go" on your dream, despite everything you should begin with something somewhat more delicate in the first place. You'll never know how things feel until you attempt it, all things considered. So if your dream includes all out accommodation, for instance, start with some light servitude or punishing, rather than a ball choke on the principal attempt.

This nice initial step can be extremely fun. An individual may make sense of another stunt is extremely fun and adds to their sexual collection, or they may learn they abhor it. In any case, information is accumulated and ideally, nobody got injured taking shape of said dream. So don't get too freeloaded out about taking things moderate.

Furthermore, regardless of whether your dream moves toward becoming something you need to seek after or not, there's no motivation to quit envisioning. There isn't just a single method to appreciate sexual dreams, Kristin Marie Bennion, authorized psychological well-being specialist, and guaranteed sex advisor tell Bustle. "A few people search out encountering the situations in their dreams, others carry on just certain perspectives, while there are numerous who are satisfied by keeping their dreams exclusively in their creative mind." And through the way toward investigating your dream, you'll make sense of what works for you.

So, what happens if you do not enjoy each other's fetish

All fetishists trust their sexual accomplices will share their enthusiasms, however, they don't depend on it. Some portion of the rush is gradually trying things out and perceiving how far they can go.

That is a significant point because gentle obsessions, for example, hitting and toe sucking, are regularly entryway practices; a method for testing an accomplice's potential responsiveness to progressively exploratory sex.

There is nothing especially surprising about that.

We live in the most explicitly dynamic period in history and the breakdown of customary limitations implies that an ever-increasing number of individuals are pushing the limits as they continued looking for sexual curiosity.

It's fine if the two accomplices are available. It's not fine if one individual is out of their customary range of familiarity and they are not confident enough to say as much.

Although you've given it each of the go and concluded that you loathe it, it is hard to connect completely in any tactile experience when there is a voice in your mind revealing to you that you feel like an imbecile.

The best way to quietness that voice is to tell your sweetheart how you feel.

He will either snicker and promise you that it doesn't make a difference, where case all your ponderousness will mystically vanish and you may find that you appreciate taking a hairbrush to his exposed base.

All fetishists trust their sexual accomplices will share their enthusiasms, yet they don't rely on it. Truth be told, some portion of the rush is gradually trying things out and perceiving how far they can go.

That is a significant point because mellow obsessions, for example, hitting and toe sucking, are regularly passage practices; a method for testing an accomplice's potential responsiveness to increasingly exploratory sex.

There is nothing especially bizarre about that.

We live in the most explicitly dynamic period in history and the breakdown of conventional limitations implies that an ever-increasing number of individuals are pushing the limits as they continued looking for sexual curiosity.

It's fine if the two accomplices are available. It's not fine if one individual is out of their customary range of familiarity and they are not emphatic enough to say as much.

Although you've given it each of them ago and concluded that you despise it, it is hard to connect completely in any tangible experience when there is a voice in your mind disclosing to you that you feel like a bonehead.

The best way to quietness that voice is to tell your sweetheart how you feel.

He will either giggle and promise you that it doesn't make a difference, where case all your clumsiness will mystically vanish and you may find that you appreciate taking a hairbrush to his uncovered base.

Or on the other hand, he won't chuckle and he won't console you, in which case you would be on the whole correct to scrutinize your long haul similarity.

Like most human conduct, fixation lies along a continuum. Toward one side are the individuals who fiddle with whips and ties.

At the opposite end are the individuals who can't engage in sexual relations without the demonstration or object that excites them.

A few specialists accept that expanded pressure, requesting lives, and higher desires are making more individuals go to sexual practices that enable them to "escape" themselves.

Fixation is by all accounts a curiously male interest.

There is no authoritative clarification for why men create sexual connections to body parts, for example, the feet and toes, however the mind area controlling the private parts is found legitimately adjacent to the cerebrum locale controlling the feet, so some kind of sign cover may clarify foot obsessions.

Likewise, delight and agony trigger the arrival of comparative synapses, for example, endorphins and serotonin and that shared trait may make disarray.

Conduct clarifications involve the relationship between being explicitly stirred and being rebuffed, and it is realized that abnormal amounts of excitement lessen the "nauseate" reaction, so novel improvements that would normally be viewed as horrendous can progress toward becoming wellsprings of sexual energy.

Fetishism is just risky on the off chance that it makes trouble the individual, or mischief to other people.

It is superbly conceivable to oblige interest inside a relationship, however just if the two accomplices can be genuine about what it intends to them.

At last, fixation is a similarly little segment of an entire relationship and long haul common sexual fulfillment is still predicated on great correspondence, an eagerness to suit each other's needs, sexual certainty, decency and the ability to regard each other's limits.

How to bring out her naughty side

Each lady can be an oddity. We likewise have terrible news: If right now in time, her wild side is as yet lying torpid, it's presumably your very own issue.

Try not to thump yourself because of all the normal sex. There is a superior sexual coexistence standing ready. Also, indeed, by better we mean a whole lot more unusual. Here's your complete manual for arousing her internal she-fallen angel. Alert, this may bring about restless evenings.

Find her fetish

Inside each lady is a sexual brute simply holding on to break free. We accept that. So chances are, on the off chance that you haven't seen her more out of control side, the issue lies with you. You should be down to calmly urge it out.

Consider wrinkles a mass of sweets in clear plastic containers. Regardless of whether you figure she doesn't have a sweet tooth, there will be one treat in the store that will roll out her improvement her brain. For most ladies, there are even a few. You must determinedly attempt them all with her. Does grimy talk leave a harsh preference for her mouth? Perhaps pretending is more her style. Possibly she feels weak at the knees over spankings. You must make sense of what her kind of decision is, and urge her to enjoy.

Alert her first

The way into a lady having a positive relationship with another sexual encounter is making her vibe protected and esteemed. Willingly volunteer to test something out without understanding her sentiments about it first, and she won't feel either. She'll feel like she's been damaged and slighted, and it won't look good for your future sexual undertakings.

If you need to accomplish something, you haven't done previously, consistently talk about it before you attempt it. It doesn't need to be an executive gathering. You can enlighten her concerning that insane move you'd like to attempt to disclose to her the amount it would turn you on, and inquire as to whether she feels good attempting it. Console her if she doesn't care for it, you'll stop, no inquiries posed. At that point, rather than having an irate lady on your hands, she's open, prepared, and willing. Unmistakably, that makes for a superior night.

Venerate her sexuality

Certainty breeds freakiness. If your lady feels compelling in her skin, and she realizes you discover every last bit of her alluring, she won't falter to place herself in under complimenting positions, attempt odd things, or contact herself before you. She'll have no questions that you're having fun.

In case you're the sort of fellow who feels awkward doling out compliments, start conveying everything that needs to be conveyed more. Try not to accept she realizes how attractive you discover her lower legs, the bend of her hips, her abdomen, her mouth—we're certain your rundown continues endlessly, simply ensure she realizes that! A confident lady is a person who will outgo and bold in bed. And keep in mind that quite a bit of that certainly ought to be natural to her, if she's inadequate with regards to, you ought to be focused on demonstrating her exactly how staggering you discover her, blemishes whatnot.

Chapter 6

Sex Tips

Men's sexual performance

You may be thinking that your performance in bed is not adequate and maybe looking for options to improve. What you should know is that you are not the only one looking for this, there are many men out there who are concerned and would want to improve their sexual performance. You may be looking for ways to satisfy your partner better while there is another man who is looking for ways to enhance his low sexual performance. You need to be aware that there are many enhancement pills available for you. You, however, do not have to visit the pharmacy or hospital if there is nothing of that attention. There are many natural ways that you can take to improve your sex life step by step. As a man, you need to be aware that your penis performs on the blood pressure, therefore your system needs to be healthy and stable. Your heart health determines your sexual health. There are many ways to keep performance high. Let us have a look.

Exercise-exercise is an important way to keep you healthy. Sex while unhealthy may cause your heart rate to go up. However, with regular exercises such as 30 minutes per day will keep you healthy and sexually active. Exercise keeps your internal organs healthy by keeping fit.

Fruits and veggies- A healthy diet is key to having a great sex life. Most importantly, it is good to have a plate that has a lot of fruits and vegetables. Some of this include

Garlic and onions-before your node at the smell, take not of the health benefits. This veges help you with proper heart circulation.

Pepper-pepper is anything chilly is important because it causes the smooth running of your blood. It further lowers the level of hypertension and inflammation of your system.

Bananas-this helps in lowering your blood pressure. Further, it helps in developing your healthy sexual organs that will aid in active sexual performance.

Food Diet-be vigilant and ensure that you take foods that have omega-three fatty acids. This includes avocado, tuna, and olive oil. This helps in increasing your blood flow. The food with vitamin B-1 is necessary for your sexual libido. These foods include kidney beans, and also pork. This kind of food sends a message to your brain that it should act fast. It sends the same message to your penis hence helping in your sexual activity. Eggs are also an important ingredient for enhancing male libido. Eggs will help in regulating your hormones such that your stress levels will go down. Stress is a contributor to low libido and sex drive.

Reduce stress

You may have experienced stress at one point in your life. You can attest that even little stress takes a toll on you and you cannot function at your full potential. That is the same thing that happens to your sexual libido when you are stressed. It goes down and there is a possibility of your hypertension going high. Stress usually increase your heartbeat which increases blood pressure and hence affects your sexual desire and libido negatively. Most of the time, when you are stressed you cannot even manage an erection. It will be a struggle because the sex drive is a mental affair. When you realize that you have a low sex drive because of stress, it would be prudent to communicate with your partner. This will help, instead of them thinking that maybe you are not interested in them anymore. While you are under stress, there are other behaviors such as drinking and smoking that may come in. This behaviors come in as a way to the cub and avoid dealing with the matter. What you do not know is that this behavior is dangerous to your sexual performance. You must see a counselor if it persists, or do everything possible to ensure that you lead a stress-free life.

Avoid unhealthy habits-What you depend on to loosen up, for example, smoking and expending liquor, could likewise influence sexual execution. While studies propose that a little red wine can improve the course, a lot of liquor can have unfriendly impacts. Stimulants tight veins and have been connected to feebleness. Chopping down or stopping smoking is one of the initial steps to improve execution. Supplanting unfortunate propensities with solid ones, for example, exercise and eating admirably can help support sexual well-being.

Vitamin D from the sun-Daylight stops the body's generation of melatonin. This hormone encourages us to rest yet additionally calms our sexual inclinations. Less melatonin implies the potential for progressively sexual want. Getting outside and giving the sun a chance to hit your skin can help wake up your sex drive, particularly throughout the winter months when the body creates more melatonin.

Practice with the masturbation-In case you're not enduring insofar as you'd like in bed, you may require some training. While sex is the most ideal approach to rehearse for sex, masturbation can likewise enable you to improve your life span. Be that as it may, how you jerk off could have adverse impacts. If you race through it, you could incidentally diminish the time you last with your accomplice. The mystery is making it last, much the same as you need to when you're not the only one.

Focus on your partner-Sex is certainly not a single direction road. Giving unique consideration to your accomplice's wants makes sex pleasurable for them, yet it can likewise help turn you on or moderate you down. Discussing this in advance can help facilitate any clumsiness if you have to back off during a hot minute. Exchanging pace or concentrating on your accomplice while you enjoy a reprieve can make for a progressively pleasant encounter for your intimacy.

Seek help-In the event that you have an erection problem, Peyronie's malady, or other analyzed issue, you may require treatment. Try to converse with your primary care physician about how you can improve your sexual presentation. It's never an awful choice to work out, eat right, and make the most of your sexual coexistence without limit.

Sex tips for couples
Extraordinary sex begins with you

Need to be great in bed? In the expressions of Rupaul, 'On the off chance that you can't love yourself, how in the damnation you going to cherish another person?' That's correct people, the key to extraordinary sex begins at home - alone!

Masturbation isn't extraordinary for finding out about your sexuality, look into recommends that independent sexual incitement diminishes pressure and reduces strain. What's more, considers have discovered that ladies who stroke off appreciate more joyful relationships, and men who discharge routinely are fundamentally more averse to create prostate malignant growth.

Praise your partner

Feeling unreliable about your room system? Odds are you're not the only one and your other half is similarly restless about their sexual mastery. Be straightforward and open with your accomplice, and disclose to them your preferences. In any case, remember to console them, so they comprehend what they're doing well (and continue doing it!)

'You can offer acclaim to your accomplice from multiple points of view, all of which help to speak with them. Positive outward appearances, nonverbal signs and verbal consolations all tally.'

'For whatever length of time that the two accomplices are fulfilled, at that point, you're having incredible sex,' she includes. 'It's the longing, or requirement for something more than breeds sexual disagreement between accomplices.'

Be real and communicate

On the off chance that you accepted the Hollywood publicity, you'd be confused with expecting amazing sex is about immediacy and energy on pianos/housetops/yachts. As a general rule, the majority of us have day employments and family duties, so insane sexploits can be hard to accomplish. However, closeness with a believed accomplice can exceed incredible sex, and you can appreciate a truly compensating sexual coexistence cuddled up at home. 'Suddenness is significant, however, it's not the most important thing in the world,' says Knight. 'Most couples, particularly those that are built up, possess little energy for without any preparation sexual encounters.' Rather, center around what works for you. If that implies heading to sleep an hour sooner on a Tuesday night for a cuddle and a spot of rumpy-pumpy, grasp it. 'It's essential to factor in a mind-blowing truth and to square with what's sensible sexual practice for you,' includes Knight. 'Getting stalled in what you "should" be doing just serves to ruin by and large sexual fulfillment.'

Try things together-While cuddling up at home has its advantages, experimentation is likewise significant, so don't be hesitant to investigate together to perceive what works for both of you. A few people love before anything else, while others just prefer to have intercourse before bed,' says Knight. 'I would state that exploring different avenues regarding various occasions isn't just fun however revives your sexual coexistence. Act naturally, be body sure, be mindful and be the test – whatever that implies for you.'

Erotic massage
How to give the best massage

If you've been needing to get your extraordinary person a loosening up back rub, read on for back rub tips that make certain to get the outcomes you need. Who doesn't love a decent knead? Getting a back rub advance unwinding, dispose of pressure and alleviate tight and sore muscles. The demonstration of rubbing likewise improves flow all through the body and depletes the lymphatic arrangement of hurtful poisons. Additionally, the private contact between a masseuse's hands and an individual's body can be amazingly erotic. If you'd like to turn out to be better versed in this craft of comprehensive mending, here are some essential back rub tips and strategies to kick you off. Your man will be in amazement of your "enchantment" fingers!

Set the Pace

Back rub is intended to unwind and de-stress along these lines, if you are giving somebody a back rub, you will need to make a feel of harmony and tranquility. Diminish the lights, play some relieving music and light scented candles around your back rub zone. Additionally, ensure the temperature in the room is marginally hotter than typical, as your accomplice will wear pretty much nothing (assuming any) dress.

It is additionally essential to utilize an appropriate back rub surface. You will require something that is firm yet agreeable and ought to be long enough to suit the full length of your accomplice. If you don't have a real back rub table, you can utilize a story tangle, bed or futon. Remember, in any case, that it is similarly significant for you to have the option to arrive at the whole zone of your accomplice's back without stressing. In this way, utilizing a couch with a high back may not be fitting on the off chance that it will hinder your entrance to the other side of your accomplice's body.

If you and your accomplice are entirely agreeable together, he will most likely need to take off his garments. You can give him a warm towel to cover his lower half during your session. On the off chance that your accomplice would prefer to wear shorts, or remain completely dressed that is OK as well.

Have your accomplice rests on the back rub surface on his stomach with his arms collapsed over his head. Ensure he is as agreeable as would be prudent. If he encounters agony or inconvenience in his lower back, neck, knees or lower legs, you can place collapsed towels or different pads underneath him as required.

You will likewise need to utilize a touch of back rub oil, for its sexy pleasure, yet more as a need. Back rub oil lessens the erosion between your hands and your accomplice's skin, which shields you from pulling the sensitive hairs on his body. You just need a modest quantity of back rub oil, so don't escape. Touch the back rub oil on your hands (not on your accomplice's skin), at that point rub your hands together for a couple of moments to make it warm.

Begin with ease

A decent back rub resembles a bit of traditional music – it begins gradually, crescendos to a peak and afterward plummets to a sensitive end. As you start your back rub, remember these essential tips.

Initially, keep one hand on your accomplice consistently. This steady contact will keep him calm and maintain a strategic distance from any astonishments during your session. Keep in mind, you need him to unwind, not ponder (or stress) about your best course of action. Second, abstain from kneading any zones with rankles, wounds or rashes. You would prefer not to disturb or spread conceivable contamination. The warm-up intends to slip your accomplice into a condition of unwinding with the goal that he can appreciate the full advantage of his back rub. Your back rub warm-up should start with a progression of smooth, musical strokes known as effleurage, a French expression signifying "to delicately contact." This method is utilized broadly during a Swedish back rub. There are a few kinds of effleurage strokes utilized at specific interims all through the back rub session. The different strokes require various measures of weight from various pieces of the hand (for instance, the fingertips or the whole palm).

Stage 1: Begin by having relaxing delicate weight with the tip of your fingers. Follow moderate, roundabout examples all over the sides of his spine. This is the place the biggest gathering of muscles in the back is found and it is likewise where you will see the most muscle hitches. If you feel a bunch in your accomplice's back, give careful consideration of its area so you can come back to it later. Move from the muscles around the spine to the shoulders, in the middle of the shoulder bones and to the neck back.

Stage 2: The next step is to apply all the more firm weight with your whole hand. Starting at the lower part of your back, gradually stroke as far as possible up to the neck, at that point right down once more. Consequently, repeat this procedure.

Stage 3: You can increase the intensity of the back rub further by utilizing just the impact point of your hand. Since you are rubbing with a littler surface zone, the weight normally increments. Apply moderate, round strokes with two hands moving outward from the upper back, at that point go up and back toward the middle. Work your direction as far as possible up to his upper back. This whole advance should take around 5 minutes.

Stage 4: After rubbing with the impact points of your hands, proceed onward to this next back rub tip. Move to the other side of your accomplice and start a more profound back rub with the tip of your fingers. Spread out your fingertips and lay one hand straightforwardly over the other so you can apply twice as much weight. Beginning at the lower back, push down solidly, moving ceaselessly from your accomplice's spine out toward his side. Daintily skim your fingers back internal and do something very similar again somewhat higher up. Stir your way up to your accomplice's upper back like this for a few minutes, at that point change to the opposite side of his body.

Presently your accomplice ought to be completely loose and prepared for the most concentrated bit of the back rub.

Go For the Deep Tissue

Because you are not an authorized proficient, you won't give a genuine profound tissue knead. Be that as it may, this is the point in your back rub session wherein you utilize the firmest measure of weight and do the most mending.

Put your hands on either side of his spine and spread out your fingers. Presently apply profound weight with your thumbs just, moving in concentric circles here and there his back. Your thumbs utilize the most grounded muscles in your grasp, and they are ideal for applying profound, extreme weight.

This is the ideal opportunity to handle any bunches you saw before. Approach these regions with increasingly delicate weight, scouring around and over the strained tissue, at that point work up to more profound weight. Check-in with your accomplice at ordinary interims to ensure that he is in no torment or uneasiness. Keep in mind, this is for his advantage.

Finish with ease

Completion with these back rub tips for a loosening up a chill off Taper the firm weight of your thumbs into a gentler manipulating by the majority of your fingers. Ply the muscles here and there your accomplice's back by copying the example a wave lapping against the shore and afterward dismantling pull out to the ocean. Following a couple of minutes, proceed onward to the strategies you utilized during the warm-up, however in the switch. Start with Step 4 and work your route in reverse to Step 1, finishing with a plume light fingertip rub.

The general intrigue of back rub isn't anything but difficult to pinpoint. Perhaps it's the incitement of muscle tissue or the moderate, concentric developments that loosen up an individual. Maybe it's the basic closeness of close human contact that makes a back rub so engaging. Whatever the explanation, the recuperating intensity of back rub is unquestionable. Utilize these back rub tips to get your man a night of arousing unwinding. Back rub is something beyond a recuperating solution for drained, throbbing muscles. A decent back rub infiltrates directly down to the spirit.

Advantages Of Erotic Massage

Note that sensual back rub is probably the most ideal approaches to unwind. Notwithstanding, a great many people don't comprehend what sensual back rub is? Be that as it may, sexual back rub includes the masseur and the collector scouring their bodies erotically and delicately. Likewise, different people may choose to utilize greasing up oil onto the body of the recipient to build up a feeling of sexual excitement. In this way, that is the reason it is imperative to recognize what is the suggestive back rub. Additionally, it is basic to know a portion of the advantages of sexual back rub before you settle on your own choice.

There is a lot of solid advantages of sensual back rub that you have to consider before you choose to utilize a suggestive back rub. On the off chance that you don't have any acquaintance with a portion of the advantages of suggestive back rub, it is prescribed that you lead your exploration.

A portion of the advantages of sensual back rub

1. Heal's muscles and joints

A suggestive back rub will assist you with improving your joint and muscle wellbeing. This is one reason why a great many people lean toward sensual back rub. With sexual back rub, it can invigorate and loosen up the muscles in your body. In this manner, if you have exhausted and hurting muscles, you are prescribed to have these sensual back rubs.

2. Enhances an erection

Note that suggestive back rub improves erections. Prostate and perineal back rubs are additionally the best to general men. Along these lines, you have to guarantee that your accomplice is gifted and ensure that the individual in question realizes how to utilize a portion of these informing fluids. It is fundamental to take note that your accomplice takes a delicate back rub.

3. Upgrades connections

On the off chance that you are seeing someone, you have to realize that sexual back rub will upgrade your relationship. Sexual back rubs are classified under erotic back rub. That is the reason most accomplices are required to attempt this kind of back rub. With this sexual back rubs, you should be cognizant and open to your feelings and emotions. This will, in this manner, advance and upgrade your relationship.

4. Forestall pressure and uneasiness

This is another advantage you are probably going to appreciate from the sexual back rub. There is a hormone in our body known as endorphin that enables the muscles to unwind after you have been needed. In this way, your accomplice has to know when you are focused and after that apply the sexual back rub to you. If the person in question does it delicately, it will diminish the feeling of anxiety in your body. Additionally, it is critical to take note of that suggestive back rub can direct the bloodstream in your body.

For the most part, this sexual back rub has numerous medical advantages. Consequently, if you have to keep up your well-being, guarantee that you practice this kind of back rub and you will encounter a lot of changes. Additionally, you may ask a specialist or a specialist to explain a portion of the issues that are confused. These, in this manner, are a snippet of data on what you have to think about sexual back rubs.

Conclusion

You have made it to the end of this book on Sex for couples, congratulations and thank you. In the book, there is an all-round discussion on what you should do to up your sex life and have a mind-blowing intimate life.

In chapter one, the book introduced you to sex and the basics of it. You learned on the importance of sex, the benefits of adopting sex communication; you were also introduced to sex stimulants. The second chapter expounded on the sex stimulants. Here, the book detailed on oral sex, oral-anal sex, foreplay, fingering, and sex toys. You got to learn the importance of stimulation before diving into sexual intercourse. The third chapter was a discussion on sex positions. You have discovered that trying out different positions helps you achieve multiple orgasms. The fourth chapter dives into the topic of sexual health. You have discovered more on physical intimacy, and also discovered the importance of sexual health. Further, the chapter has dived into Anal sex and given you all the details that you need to know before you engage in anal sex. The fifth chapter has talked about sexual fantasy. Everyone has a fantasy. You have learned how to bring out the naughty side of your partner and how to solve fetish problems. The sixth and final chapter has discussed on the tips that you should note as a couple. The book has discussed the health benefits that will keep your libido up, as well as sex tips for couples. Further, the chapter gives you some amazing tips on giving your partner an erotic. Finally, if you found this book useful in any way, a review on Amazon is always appreciated!